The
No-Drugs Guide
to Better Health

by

Eleonore Blaurock-Busch, Ph.D.

with

Bernd W. Busch, M.S., D.C.

Parker Publishing Company, Inc.
West Nyack, New York

© 1984 by

Eleonore Blaurock-Busch

West Nyack, N.Y.

Library of Congress Cataloging in Publication Data

Blaurock-Busch, Eleonore.
  The no-drugs guide to better health.

  Includes bibliographies and index.
  1. Naturopathy. 2. Therapeutics—Popular works.
I. Busch, Bernd W. II. Title.
RZ440.B56 1984   615.5'35   83-13195

ISBN 0-13-623090-3
ISBN 0-13-623082-2 {PBK}

Printed in the United States of America

Dedication

To my parents who built the foundation, to my husband for his advice and support, to my children for their understanding and willingness to share, to Ilse Nürnberger and all the wonderful teachers in my life, to Florence Becker Lennon who made this all possible by teaching me "chutzpah," and last but not least, to all the people worldwide who recognize the importance of natural health care.

Acknowledgments

Special thanks to *Bestways* magazine for permission to use material published in my column, "Eleonore's Herbals" from that magazine in this book.

How These Remedies Can Help You

This book is not anti-medicine, and my aim is not to persuade you to ignore medical advice. Instead, I hope to encourage you to be realistic about all healing methods and to use common sense when choosing health care treatments. Learn to listen to your body and give natural remedies a try first. Why ask for a Librium prescription when a cup of valerian tea can be more beneficial? Why pop antacids when cabbage juice can soothe an irritated stomach and quickly heal peptic ulcers? The truth is that many times a simple, inexpensive remedy improves your condition as quickly and as effectively as drugs, without causing dangerous side effects. While drugs seem to provide fast relief, they often induce other, more complex, health problems or actually worsen the condition you are trying to cure.

Give natural healing methods a chance. The old-time remedies discussed in this book are an alternative to drug therapy. They are simple and inexpensive and they have withstood the test of time. Most of all, they are effective and harmless.

Today, every parent worries about drug abuse but rarely realizes that drug abuse starts long before Valium or heroin addiction. How many of today's parents think nothing of administering painkillers to a cranky, yet healthy infant? I once had a neighbor who gave aspirin to her three-year-old every time the little girl refused to take her nap, and this young mother found it rather odd that I preferred a tired, irritable youngster to a drugged one. Besides, a warm cup of fennel or camomile tea sweetened with a touch of honey does induce sleep equally well.

Considering natural remedies first could quickly reduce drug abuse and dependency. While drug therapy and surgery are excellent emergency treatments, they do not have to be our one and only choice of treatments.

In Europe, natural remedies are part of the health care system. Health spa officials and physicians continue to endorse and prescribe them as they have for centuries. Germany's national health care insurance covers a variety of natural therapies, and consequently, natural remedies are treated with respect. Many doctors continue to consider natural remedies first.

Every year, millions of Germans seek natural treatments. If these often old-fashioned remedies did not effectively relieve suffering, Germany's government officials would think twice before endorsing their use.

Read this book and give old-time remedies a try. Many of these simple and inexpensive remedies have helped people for centuries and will, most likely, be of use to you. Read this book carefully; it can be your passport to good health.

—*Eleonore Blaurock-Busch, Ph.D.*

Foreword

"Why take Librium when a cup of valerian tea can be more beneficial?" asks Eleonore Blaurock-Busch in this wisdom-filled book. For that matter, why not consider chicken soup instead of antibiotics, thyme rather than penicillin, cabbage juice for peptic ulcer instead of Tagamet, eucalyptus oil instead of Dristan, peppermint tea rather than Bendectin, rosmarin leaves instead of Motrin and other anti-arthritics, chiropractic manipulation instead of cortisone, cherry juice rather than Zyloprim for gout, celery instead of Diuril, acupuncture rather than chemical analgesics, garlic instead of the anti-hypertensive Inderal, and shave grass rather than tetracycline for acne?

Practically every American will immediately recognize the trade name products in the preceding paragraph, but how many have even a superficial acquaintance with yarrow sitz baths, fennel tea, loofah sponges, poultices, fomentations, or vapor baths?

In her dedication, Eleonore Blaurock-Busch, Ph.D., expresses gratitude to the person who taught her "chutzpah," a word—no, a concept—that may require translation for those of you who are not Jewish or familiar with the idiom of New York's Broadway. The simple words "nerve" or "gall" or "arrogance" fail to transmit the flavor of chutzpah. This word/concept, which is rapidly becoming an integral part of the English language, is best exemplified by the child who kills both his parents and then pleads for mercy on the grounds that he is now an orphan.

Dr. Blaurock-Busch demonstrates this remarkable quality of chutzpah—this combination of courage and audacity—when she prescribes traditional remedies in this era of modern medicine, when she recommends Old World treatments to a New World audience, when she emphasizes the historical to a generation taught to worship the contemporary. Yet, with talent and charm, she achieves her goal in such a comprehensive, elegant, thoroughly documented, easily readable manner that she deserves the highest accolade—"chutzpah cum laude."

The reader can use the book as a reference and look up any disease—from scoliosis to sciatica, diabetes to dental caries, hypoglycemia to herpes, kidney stones to cataracts—and many other conditions. Or,

7

the reader can use the book for its sage beauty advice for skin, hair, nails and teeth, or for its practical and conservative approach to sports injuries and first aid. Or, the reader can, as I did, read the book from cover to cover and learn how to avoid the dark country of modern medicine and, with the invaluable help of this "passport to good health," enter a new, exciting, optimistic land of personal responsibility, independence, and long life.

Robert S. Mendelsohn, M.D.

December 1982

Comment

I am happy that you are helping your readers find the natural way to health and healthy living.

At the turn of this century, my father, Dr. Max Bircher-Benner, discovered new avenues to health care, and he fought hard to make them available to all people. The success of his clinic, founded in 1904 in Zurich, proved that he was right.

During the thirty years of my association with his clinic, I was able to witness how this approach was of benefit to many people.

I am pleased that you, in your own way, also aim to, and actually do help your readers, and I wish your book great success.

Yours,

Ruth Kunz-Bircher

Table of Contents

and Old Ways to Control Colic • Proven European Herbal Tea Mixtures that Strengthen Your Stomach • Simple Home Treatments for Colitis • Gypsy Remedies and Other Ancient Treatments That Overcome Constipation • Inexpensive Kneipp Remedies for Hemorrhoids • My Parents' Secret Home Remedy That Quickly Stops Diarrhea • Asian and European Folk Treatments that Control and Prevent Intestinal Bacteria • How the Bulgarians Prevent Digestive Disorders

Some Facts About Arthritis • Ancient Arthritic Remedies from Around the World • How the Europeans Approach Arthritis • Another Old-Fashioned Herbal Remedy for Arthritic Pain • How the Romans Eased Arthritic Pain • How Spinal Manipulation Helps Relieve Arthritic Misery • Relieving Pain with Chinese Remedies • An Old-Fashioned Diet for Gout • Coping with Osteoporosis • Preventing Backaches with Simple Exercises • Helpful Hints for Sciatica • Controlling Scoliosis • Food and Herbs for Healthy Bones

Improving Your Lifestyle • Lifestyle Quiz • German Researchers Endorse Herbal Treatment for Liver Diseases Including Hepatitis and Jaundice • Useful Folk Remedies for Fatty Liver Disease and Cirrhosis • Old-Time Water Treatments That Stimulate Liver Function • Money-Saving Home Remedies for Liver and Gallbladder Ailments • Simple Herbal Treatments for Dyspepsia and Gallbladder Problems • An Ancient Remedy that Stimulates the Flow of Bile (or How to Live Without a Gallbladder) • Preventing Gallbladder Colic, the Old-Fashioned Way • An Updated Customary Diet Plan That Reduces Cholesterol • Traditional Herbal Remedies That Strengthen Your Heart • Natural Treatments for Kidney Ailments • Herbal Juices That Strengthen Bladder and Kidney • Avoiding Kidney Stones • Traditional Remedies for Urinary Infections • Natural Diuretics

for Herpes Infections and Skin Eruptions • Reducing "Old-
Age Spots" • Preventing and Treating Wrinkles • Aiding Sun-
burn • Easy Ways to Correct Excessive Sweating and Body
Odors • Your Nails Reveal Your State of Health • Grandma's
Remedy for Brittle Eyelashes • Customary European Treat-
ments for Healthier Hair

Healthy Teeth for a Lifetime • My Father's Old-Time Dental
Products • Traditional Recipes for Homemade Toothpaste •
European Tooth Powders for Sparkling Teeth • Easy-to-Make
Old-Country Mouthwashes and Gargles • Old-World Reme-
dies for Toothaches • European Teething Aid for Infants •
What to Do About Thrush • Ancient Ways to Control Gum
Problems • Old Herbal Remedies for Mouth Ulcers and
Canker Sores • Freshen Your Breath, Naturally

How I Eased My Daughter's Earache • Fighting Infections with
an Old-Fashioned Antibiotic • Special Tips for Controlling
Nosebleeds • How to Deal with Plugged Nasal Passages • Help-
ing Allergies and Sinusitis—the Traditional Way • Natural
Methods for Better Eyesight • Healthy Foods for Healthy Eyes
• Correcting Night Blindness and Other Visual Problems •
Simple Remedies for Glaucoma • Combining Old and New
Treatments to Relieve Cataracts

You and Sports • Preventing Sports Injuries • Emergency Care
for the Seriously Injured • When and How to Take Care of
Minor Injuries • Treating Strains • Quick Self-Help for Sprains
• Simple European Remedies Prevent and Relieve Muscle
Soreness and Other Athletic Injuries • Folk Healers' Remedy
for Bruises • Improving Low Back Pain • Taking Care of Torn
Cartilage • Coping with Leg Cramps • Overcoming Runners'

Aches and Pains • Traditional Remedies for Sensible Foot
Care • Useful Remedies that Remove Calluses, Corns and
Bunions • Simple Treatment for Frostbites

Cancer—What Causes It? • Reducing the Cancer Risk • Looking at an Old-Wives' Tale • Natural Cancer Therapies • Helping Cystic Fibrosis • An Unconventional Treatment for Cerebral Palsy • Century-Old Remedies that Improve Parkinson's
Disease (*Paralysis Agitans*) • Old-Fashioned Dry Brush Massage
• Selecting the Right Kind of Doctor • Accepting Responsibilities • Natural Healing Guide

1

Fighting Off Colds and Flus
with Traditional Old Country Remedies

MY FAMILY'S SENSIBLE APPROACH TO NATURAL
HOME REMEDIES

I grew up in drugstores, yet I can easily count the number of aspirins or any such painkiller that I have taken in the forty-two years of my life. Sure, I occasionally suffer from colds or headaches, but when this happens, I try natural remedies first. It's simpler and less troublesome.

I am scared of drugs. I have seen too many people who started out with a simple headache or a case of nervous tension who wound up drug-dependent. I have also spoken with people of all ages who expected miracles from medicine and found much-needed help from simple old-time remedies.

My parents had three drugstores (one for each child) and though I remember neatly stacked bottles and pills, my earliest memories are of herbal teas, tinctures, and extracts. We always had a pot of herbal tea sitting on the stove and I can think of many occasions when our family doctor stopped in to have a cup of tea and to discuss methods of treatment.

In Germany, drugstores are different from "apothecaries." While the latter handle mainly prescription drugs, drugstores are health-oriented. Over-the-counter pharmaceuticals are sold, but the main emphasis remains on natural remedies. Druggists used to make anything from shoe polish, paint and rat poison to natural cough remedies and actually prepared these products in their own stores. I do remember watching my father make arthritic ointments and other natural products, but today's German druggists hardly prepare anything. Instead, products are manufactured by major pharmaceutical companies who think nothing of supplying and promoting natural *and* pharmaceutical products.

During my early childhood, however, drugs were a rarity. Whatever medication was available was used for emergencies. Doctors had to promote natural remedies because there simply was no other choice. I never received antibiotics although I had plenty of sore throats.

"Have her drink hot marshmallow or thyme tea, let her gargle with salt water, thyme or camomile tea, and put her to bed. Promote sweating and when she feels hungry have her eat vegetable soup." Such was our doctor's advice.

It might very well have saved my life. At age eighteen I came down with meningitis and when I received my first antibiotic treatment I quickly responded. Who knows what would have happened had I received antibiotics many times before. Penicillin immunity, which has now become a reality, was unheard of twenty years ago.

My parents always enforced natural remedies. I have never taken synthetic laxatives or any other drug for that matter. I have learned to eat high-roughage foods like beets and whole-grain bread (Vollkornbrot) long before nutritionists realized the importance of such foods. In severe cases of constipation, I had to drink father's special herbal laxative tea that always worked wonders and never created dependency.

I also learned to endure a certain amount of pain. Children's aspirin simply did not exist. We drank witch hazel tea for minor headaches before we were sent to bed. For a toothache mother applied her special poultice or clove oil.

It was all rather simple and it worked. Today, I soothe my family's aches and pains pretty much the way my mother did and I have yet to encounter a situation that these old-time remedies could not handle successfully.

HOW GRANDMA COPED WITH THE COMMON COLD

When we were irritable, nervous, or depressed, we received hugs and encouragement instead of drugs.

Grandma knew cold symptoms all too well and whenever we displayed signs such as fatigue, plus a runny nose, a cough, or a fever, we were immediately put on her "cold therapy."

Grandma swore that thyme tea quickly eliminated cold symptoms. She was right. Today, research indicates that the herb thyme (*Thymus vulgaris*) effectively relieves simple coughs, bronchitis, and laryngitis. Thyme is also an effective antibiotic and antispasmodic and has been found useful for spastic coughs such as whooping cough and asthma. Thyme's main ingredient is thymol, a strong antiseptic that is 25 times more effective than phenol. Other important ingredients of garden thyme or wild thyme (*Thymus serpyllum*), also called mother of thyme, are its aromatic oils, carvacrol plus tannin, and antibiotic substances. Thyme helps to expel gas and has been found useful for chronic gastritis. It certainly aids all respiratory problems. Thyme is listed in the German pharmacopoeia.

Children should be given 2–3 cups of thyme tea per day. Adults can take more. In addition, 4–6 drops of arnica tincture should be added to each cup of tea, depending on age. Adults should take 6–8 drops. Arnica (*Arnica montana*) stimulates the metabolism, thus helping to overcome fatigue.

In the evenings, Grandma recommended one cup of her special herbal tea mixture consisting of equal parts of black elder flowers (*Sambuccus nigra*), coltsfoot (*Tussilago farfara*), lance-leaf plantain (*Plantago lanceolato*), German camomile (*Matricaria chamomilla*) and linden flowers (*Tilia europaea or T. americana*), sweetened with a touch of honey. This tea helps to eliminate cold symptoms and provides a restful sleep.

Alternating footbaths were used to stimulate the body's immune system. This simple Kneipp therapy is still part of European spa treatments and is easily administered. During my childhood, two small buckets were filled with water, one ice-cold, the other hot. We always had to start out with the hot water, alternating back and forth for about ten minutes. You can use your bathtub instead. Sit on the edge of your tub and have hot water running over your feet until it feels uncomfortable, which is after about 1–2 minutes. Switch to cold water for another 1–2 minutes and keep switching several times. This old-fashioned remedy stimulates circulation, relieves nasal catarrh, and improves tension and migraine headaches. One word of caution, though. Alternating baths should *never* be used by people suffering from varicose veins as this causes veins to dilate.

When we felt sick, we were sent to bed and all we got to eat was some vegetable soup, because Grandma believed that cold sufferers needed fluids more than solid food, a view that is now shared by numerous European health care practitioners.

Juices made from carrots, grapes, oranges, or lemons were also part of Grandma's "cold therapy" which, of course, supplied plenty of needed vitamins and minerals. Carrot juice, for instance, is rich in vitamin A (one medium carrot supplies 5,000 International Units), which is the nutrient that helps to fight infections. Grapes, lemons, and oranges are all rich in vitamin C, and while these juices are good sources of natural nutrients, it is my experience that additional vitamin C (500 to 1000 mg every hour) speeds up recovery.

CONTROLLING FEVER

Fever is the body's natural response to infection. It is a defense mechanism that alerts and actually mobilizes your immune system to fight whatever invades and threatens your system. Functionally, fever is caused by a disruption of the normal heat regulating mechanism. Causes are infections, trauma, injury, or dehydration. Fever can be produced by drugs and cause a vicious cycle of heat production which may terminate in heat stroke. The higher the fever, the faster the pulse rate. Fever also speeds up breathing and causes fatigue. While temperatures of above 103 degrees Fahrenheit may induce convulsions, serious cell damage usually begins when the body temperature rises above 106 degrees Fahrenheit. When the fever rises to 110 degrees F., the person usually has only a few hours to live unless his temperature is rapidly brought back within normal range by sponging the patient's body with alcohol, which evaporates and cools the body, or by bathing in ice water.

Most fevers, however, fluctuate between 100 and 102 degrees Fahrenheit, and the body seems to have a built-in thermostat that prevents extreme high fevers. In fact, people rarely suffer from fever that exceeds 106 degrees.

During a recent conference I talked with Dr. Herbert Lee from Toronto, Canada, about old-fashioned fever treatments and Dr. Lee revealed how he had once used a traditional treatment to relieve his young daughter's high fever.

"We did what our parents and yesterday's doctors used to do," he said. "We applied cold compresses. It helped, but she still ran a high fever and experienced convulsions. We then prepared a bath of cold water and simply immersed her body. It helped. Her fever dropped almost instantly and the convulsions stopped."

Prior to the outbreak of fever, people often feel shaky and cold, a sensation that is followed by an outbreak of sweating. This is, of course, a warning that should not be ignored. It is the brain's way of telling the body to turn on its furnace to raise body temperature to a higher setting. This sensation of coldness also signals to the person that additional support is needed. Warm clothes, blankets, and the drinking of liquids all help to raise body temperature, which in turn aids and accelerates the body's defense mechanism.

Black elder tea (*Sambuccus nigra*) sweetened with a little honey has been used for centuries to reduce fever in people suffering from colds and flu. Another herbal remedy that has been found useful and is still recommended by German health care practitioners is a mixture of:

> arnica flowers (*Arnica montana*)
> black elder (*Sambuccus nigra*)
> buck bean (*Menyanthes trifoliata*)
> butterwort (also called yellow gentian root) (*Gentiana lutea*)
> willow bark (*Salix alba*)
>
> Use 2 teaspoons of herbal tea mixture per 1 pint water. Bring to quick boil, remove from heat and steep for 5 minutes. Take 1–3 cups in small doses throughout the day.

Feverish patients should rest and drink plenty of fluids to prevent dehydration. In addition to the herbal teas outlined above, juices should be supplied generously. Beet juice has been found to be especially valuable. It is rich in nutrients, especially vitamins A and C, and does not upset the stomach.

Applying cold compresses to the forehead and neck areas comforts the patient and reduces fever. Cold compresses wrapped around the forearms and calves also help to bring down temperature; however, the key to fever treatment is aiding the body in reducing its temperature output. Cooling the skin is one way of doing just that. Drinking plenty of liquids prevents dehydration.

Feverish patients don't appreciate overheated rooms, thus German doctors generally recommend that room temperature does not exceed 60 to 65 degrees Fahrenheit. Fresh air aids recuperation, but drafts should, of course, be avoided. In addition, it is best to keep patients in a room that has subdued lighting and provides a relaxing atmosphere.

Fever should not be regarded as a threat to health because it activates the immune system by stimulating the production of a certain type of white blood cells, called monocytes, that actually engulf foreign invaders like viruses, bacteria, fungi, allergens, and even certain drugs.

Generally, people's fear of fever is unjustified, and new research seriously questions the use of fever-reducing drugs such as aspirin and amphetamines for fevers below 104 degrees Fahrenheit. Dr. Matthew J. Kluger, psychologist at the Michigan Medical School and author of *Fever: Its Biology, Evolution and Function,* published by Princeton University Press, is one of the leading researchers of fever therapy. He and other physicians, including pediatricians, support the old theory which suggests that fever should be allowed to run its course since it may actually shorten illness.

In addition, studies at the University of Texas Health Science Center in Dallas indicate that fever supports antibiotic therapy, and researchers at Yale University School of Medicine demonstrated that fever helps to contain infections and actually reduces the chance of spreading the infection to others. Contrary to people's belief feverish patients are less contagious than those who suffer from the same infection but suppress their fever with medication.

So don't reach for fever-reducing drugs every time you are running a temperature. Give your body a chance to heal itself. As Thomas Sydenham, the seventeenth-century English physician said, "Fever is Nature's engine which she brings into the field to remove her enemy."

RELIEVING BRONCHIAL COUGHS AND ASTHMA WITH INEXPENSIVE HOT PACKS AND VAPOR BATHS

For centuries, heat has been known to aid respiratory ailments. Herbal poultices (also called cataplasms) and vapor baths have been part of health care since ancient days. The Egyptians used these remedies, as did the Aztecs, the Indians, and the Chinese, all of whom had a highly developed knowledge of herbal medicine.

Hot herbal packs and vapor baths supply the respiratory tract with moist heat and healing substances such as alkaloids that are known to reduce pain. Azulene, another herbal ingredient, soothes irritated and inflamed membranes. Herbal expectorants such as fennel seeds (*Foeniculum vulgare*) or lungwort (*Pulmonaria officinalis*) promote the discharge of mucus from the respiratory passages, and herbal antispasmodics such as linden flowers (*Tilia europaea or T. americana*) help to prevent asthma attacks. As I have pointed out before, thyme (*Thymus vulgaris*) has antibiotic properties and benefits all infectious respiratory ailments.

To prepare a herbal poultice, brush or bruise herb, moisten with hot water and spread mixture on wet, hot cloth. Apply to chest or back (lung area) and remove when cold. After treatment, wash area with camomile infusion.

Fomentations are a similar and somewhat simpler form of hot packs. To make them, soak cloth or towel in an herbal infusion or decoction, wring out excess, and apply to affected area. Remove when cold.

For an inhalant vapor bath you need a chair, a towel, and a pot containing a steaming herbal infusion. Sit on chair and hold your head over the steaming pot, drape towel to contain vapors, and inhale for as long as it feels comfortable, which is around 10 to 15 minutes.

Asthma attacks can be prevented with hot packs when combined with hot foot or hand baths. This traditional emergency treatment continues to be used by European health care practitioners who also recommend that asthma and bronchitis sufferers eat a salt-free vegetarian diet. Fresh fruits and vegetables are to be preferred to cooked foods. A cup of valerian tea (*Valeriana officinalis*) taken before bedtime will provide a restful sleep.

MEDICINAL HERBS FOR HOT PACKS AND VAPOR BATHS

anise seeds (*Pimpinella anisum*)

althea root (*Althaea officinalis*)

camomile (*Matricaria chamomilla*)

coltsfoot (*Tussilago farfara*)

fennel seeds (*Foeniculum vulgare*)

Iceland moss (*Lichen islandicus*)

linden flowers or bark (*Tilia europaea* or *T. americana*)

thyme (*Thymus vulgaris*)

violet leaves (also called pansy) (*Viola tricolor*)

FATHER'S SIMPLE RECIPES FOR COUGH DROPS AND SYRUPS

Cough drops and syrups don't have to contain artificial colors, flavors, and preservatives. They can be just as tasty, appealing, and effective if made from natural ingredients only.

While in Germany recently, I visited drugstores and I certainly noticed changes, though natural products like father used to prepare still dominate the market. Natural fennel syrup, anise, fennel, and eucalyptus cough drops continue to be big sellers with the only difference being that these old-time cold remedies are now produced and marketed by big companies.

Try the following old-fashioned recipes and you will be well prepared for the next cold season.

Natural Cough Syrups

Mix 3 oz. honey, add 6 drops of fennel oil (or 3 drops fennel oil and 3 drops anise oil). Shake well and store.

or

Take 1 oz. of fennel seed, ground, and 4 oz. of honey. Combine in a small saucepan and bring to boil. Filtering would eliminate cloudiness, but is not necessary.

Cough Drops

10 oz. light-brown sugar
3 oz. water, plus
20 drops fennel oil or extract, or
10 drops fennel oil or extract plus 10 drops of anise oil, or
20 drops of wintergreen extract (*Gaultheria procumbens*), or
20 drops of eucalyptus extract (*Eucalyptus globulus*) depending on taste.

Add all ingredients into pot and bring to a slow boil. Continue to simmer for approximately 20 minutes. Use spoon to test for consistency by dipping into boiling syrup.

Remove and dip into cold water to test for hardness. Cough drops are done when syrup hardens quickly in cold water and is not soft to touch.

Pour mixture onto well-greased cookie sheet and let cool. Cough drops should be cut before completely hardened, or can be broken in pieces when cold.

Undercooked cough drops will continue to be sticky even when cold. Overcooked candies, however, will be porous instead of clear and crystalline. If either one happens, simply heat up mixture again and start over.

Recently, I was invited to appear on a Denver TV talk show to reminisce about some of these traditional remedies my father passed on to me. Prior to the show, I prepared all sorts of cough remedies and did come up with nice samples of fennel cough syrup, as well as anise, fennel, and wintergreen cough drops. I poured the syrup into attractive bottles, placed the odd-shaped cough drops in crystal bowls, and showed it all on the air. The response was fantastic. Some people called the station, a good number kept our office phone busy, and an overwhelming number contacted me through *Bestways* magazine. Actually, the letters I receive on a daily basis indicate that there is a growing demand for natural remedies, and I do appreciate this promising trend in health care.

Another old-fashioned yet effective cough syrup is made from onions and honey. It's my mother-in-law's speciality. If you like onions, give this remedy a try. It is an effective expectorant. In addition, onions have antiseptic, antispasmodic, stomachic, and tonic properties and have long been recognized to be useful medicinally.

Onion and Honey Cough Syrup

Cut up 6 white onions and put in pot. Add ½ cup raw honey and cook over low heat for 2 hours. Take warm in small doses throughout the day.

HOW GRANDPA HANDLED LARYNGITIS AND HOARSENESS

Any heat treatment benefits laryngitis and hoarseness and reduces discomfort.

My grandfather believed in hot milk and honey, though he modified this old remedy by adding one teaspoon of fennel cough syrup to one cup of hot milk. This reduces inflammation, helps relieve flatulence, and promotes a restful sleep.

Grandpa's tasty herbal tea mixture, another modified, traditional remedy, can easily be prepared at home.

Herbal Tea for Laryngitis and Hoarseness

Mix 1 oz. of althea root (*Althaea officinalis*)
1 oz. of licorice root (*Glycyrrhiza glabra*)
1 oz. of coltsfoot (*Tussilago farfara*)
½ oz. of mullein (*Verbascum nigrum*)
½ oz. of pimpernel (*Pimpinella saxifraga*)
Steep 1 tsp. in 1 cup boiling-hot water. Sweeten with honey and drink hot, 2–4 cups per day.

Gargling with a hot camomile infusion (1 teaspoon herb to 1 cup water) soothes irritated membranes.

WHAT TO DO ABOUT NASAL CATARRH

A stuffy nose is worse than a runny one, and modern treatment seems to be limited to nasal sprays, and, if you live in a dry climate, the use of humidifiers. While the latter help to relieve discomfort, you can improve a humidifier's action by adding two or three drops of eucalyptus oil to the water, but be sure that your humidifier is suited for this. If not, simply add a few drops of eucalyptus oil to a pot of boiling water and simmer on your stove. Eucalyptus oil's unique scent will soon fill the air and open nasal passages.

A vapor bath using eucalyptus oil (*Eucalyptus globulus*), peppermint oil (*Mentha piperita*), or camomile (*Matricaria chamomilla*) relieves congestion quickly. (Review "Relieving bronchial cough and asthma with inexpensive hot packs and vapor baths" earlier in this chapter.)

There is another effective natural treatment that quickly relieves nasal congestion and that is sniffing water. Try it. It works.

Have you ever noticed that a stuffy nose is more bothersome at night and that symptoms improve after you have been up and around for a few hours? Dr. Paul M. Seebohm, author of *Family Practice* says exercise reverses the congestive effect of rhinitis, also called "stuffy nose." Dr. Seebohm demonstrated that a vigorous three-minute exercise program promotes beneficial responses that are better than those seen in patients treated with chemical decongestants.

Vitamin C is known to have antihistamine properties, thus it is useful in treating nasal congestion due to hay fever and sinusitis. Vitamin C does not cause drowsiness, instead, it can help you feel better. Take 500–1000 mg every hour to relieve discomfort.

OVERCOMING HEADACHES AND MUSCLE TENSION

Headache, an almost universal complaint, may not be considered a disabling ailment, but a splitting headache certainly limits any individual's efficiency. As Cervantes wrote in *Don Quixote*, "When the head aches, all the body is out of tune." Thomas Jefferson complained, "An attack of the periodical head-ache ... came on me about a week ago rendering me unable as yet either to write or read without great pain."

While tension, fatigue, frustration, anxiety, even resentment are often the underlying causes of headaches, Dr. Seymour Diamond, assistant professor of neurology, the Chicago Medical School, describes three basic categories of headaches.

1. *Vascular headaches* are due to dilation (swelling) of blood vessels in the head and may be caused by food additives such as nitrates, or MSG (Monosodium glutamate), or drugs.

2. *Muscle tension headaches* are due to tightening of head and neck muscles and their underlying causes are most often tension, fatigue, and depression. Muscle tension headaches can also be brought on by excessive eye strain.

3. *Headaches due to organic problems* are brought on by problems such as injuries, infections, inflammation of the brain lining, and brain tumors. Headaches of that nature are generally ac-

companied by a number of specific symptoms and need to be treated accordingly.

"Treatment of headache depends on the cause," says Dr. Jack Antel, assistant professor of neurology at the University of Chicago. Headaches due to muscle tension are quickly relieved by relaxing tense muscles. A warm camomile poultice followed by a gentle massage using pine needle oil or peanut oil often reduces headaches and muscle tension. Manipulation or acupuncture are other classic and successful therapies.

In Europe, pine needle extract is widely used to relax muscle strains and pains.

Pine Needle Extract

To make pine needle extract, add 3 oz. young pine needle shoots to 6 oz. ethanol. Let soak for 8 days and filter. Rub extract onto painful areas.

This old-fashioned rubbing, now exquisitely packaged, can still be found in German drugstores. It continues to be my mother's main headache and muscle tension treatment. If that doesn't work, a chiropractic adjustment generally relieves discomfort quickly.

Headaches can also be caused by nutritional deficiencies. Anemia is a common cause of headache, but by supplying your diet with iron and other needed nutrients you may remove symptom and cause.

Stress-induced headaches also respond favorably to vitamin therapy. Vitamin B complex for instance, commonly referred to as the "stress vitamin," is known to reduce tension headaches.

Lori M. frequently suffered from excruciating headaches that became particularly severe during her menstrual period. A nutritional deficiency test suggested multiple nutritional deficiencies. Subsequently, a blood analysis was ordered and an iron deficiency (anemia) was revealed. Lori started to take chelated iron plus a vitamin B-complex and other nutritional supplements, and soon started to feel better. Manipulation and massage provided relief from pain, and in time, her headaches disappeared altogether.

MOTHER'S SECRET REMEDIES FOR SORE THROAT AND "STREP" THROAT

Sore throats are as common among children as bruises and cuts are, and if accompanied by a mild fever they are capable of putting mothers in a state of frenzy. "Strep" is feared, and the general approach is to call the pediatrician. A "strep" test is then scheduled, and many times antibiotics are given long before results are conclusive. This sort of drug abuse now concerns many people as it has led to a growing "antibiotic immunity" among America's youngsters.

Streptococcal infection can lead to complications such as rheumatic fever and therefore, treatment is necessary; however, antibiotics should *never* be given unless laboratory results are clearly positive. While it is true that streptococcus infection is commonplace among children, it is not as prevalent as is feared and suggested.

Parents need to be good detectives, and that is particularly true when it comes to childhood diseases. Identifying ailments and evaluating symptoms helps to prevent panicky situations and can do wonders for your pocketbook. Why spend money for doctor bills and prescription items when simple remedies can help equally well? Besides, old-fashioned natural remedies make excellent emergency treatments that can be helpful until laboratory tests are conclusive.

During my childhood, "strep throat" was as prevalent as it is today, yet antibiotic therapy was seldom used. Whatever antibiotics were available were used up quickly in army hospitals to treat emergencies, and there were plenty of those. Naturally, well-meaning, concerned family doctors could not have administered antibiotics even if they had wanted to. The supply was too limited and general practitioners had to make use of alternative treatments.

I have to give credit to my mother and the many parents and grandparents of that time for their common-sense approach. Often, during an air raid, they had to take the initiative and accept responsibility during emergencies when doctors were kept away by bombings, fire, or emergency surgery. Many people's lives were saved by an attentive, knowledgeable mother who simply remembered when and how to apply natural remedies.

The following treatment was my mother's standard treatment for sore and "strep" throat—and our family doctor endorsed and prescribed it with confidence.

TREATMENT FOR SORE AND "STREP" THROAT

1. Bed rest if patient is feverish
2. Gargle with:
   hot diluted lemon juice, or
   hot salt water, or

hot camomile tea (M. *chamomilla*), or

hot althea root tea (*Althaea officinalis*), or

hot infusion of equal parts of mallow leaves (*Malva sylvestris*), mullein (*Verbascum thapsus*), and Iceland moss (*Cetraria islandica*).

Use: soak in cold water for 1–2 hours, bring to short boil. Strain and use hot.

3. Drink 3 cups of the following herbal tea mixture daily:

   2 parts of Iceland moss (*C. islandica*), one of nature's best antibiotics.

   2 parts of coltsfoot (*Tussilago farfara*)

   1 part of garden cress (*Lepidium sativum*).

   This herbal tea has excellent antibiotic and astringent properties.

4. Nutritional supplements to be taken daily:

   15 grains of garlic oil (*Allium sativum*) 6 times daily. Garlic is one of the best natural antibiotics and antiseptics, and it does reduce fever, however, if it causes gastric problems, stay away from it.

   500 mg vitamin C every hour (adults can take more). During illness, particularly infections, there seems to be an increased demand for this vitamin. Therefore, it is best to supply it throughout the day. When the body's need for vitamin C has been met, signs of diarrhea may occur. Discontinuing the vitamin plus eating a slice of slightly burned toast quickly eliminates the problem (see Chapter 2).

   10,000 International Units (I.U.) of vitamin A twice daily. (Adults: 50,000 I.U. daily.) Patients often ask me about vitamin A toxicity and I generally point out that this "vitamin A phobia" is hardly justified. Toxicity has occurred in adults who have taken 100,000 to 500,000 units for over 15 months or longer, and toxicity signs such as loss of hair, sore lips, flaky itching skin, painful joints, and tenderness and swelling over the long bones disappeared within a few days after the vitamin had been discontinued. No fatalities have ever been reported.

5. Applying a throat poultice relieves discomfort quickly. Use a clean towel, soak in warm camomile infusion, apply to throat, and leave on until cold. Repeat if necessary.

6. Wash feverish patient with lukewarm vinegar water (three spoons vinegar to two pints water). This favorite Kneipp therapy has been found useful in reducing fever. A vinegar-water compress applied around the legs and arms can be used instead.

7. Juice fasting is recommended until fever is reduced to nearly normal. Juices should be supplied generously and the first solid foods eaten should be fresh fruits and vegetables.

MOTHER'S WAY OF DEALING WITH WHOOPING COUGH

The first signs of a rough, hacking cough were warning signals to Mother and escaping her treatment was like escaping from Sing Sing.

To relieve coughing, she prepared her special tea mixture of sage (*Salvia officinalis*), anise seed (*Anisum sativum*), primrose (*Primula officinalis*), althea root (*Althaea officinalis*), elder flowers (*Sambuccus nigra*), thyme (*Thymus vulgaris*) and violet (*Viola odorato*). A touch of honey was added to each cup of tea. Children had to drink two cups a day.

Her onion cough syrup (see "Father's simple recipes for cough drops and syrups" earlier in this chapter) had to be taken faithfully every hour on the hour and before bedtime, and a cup of valerian tea (*Valeriana officinalis*) taken before bedtime insured a restful night.

To the vapor bath she added a few drops of her special herbal oil mixture. It consisted of:

5 parts of eucalyptus oil
5   "   of pine needle oil
5   "   of camphor oil
1   "   of clove oil.

Mother also believed in the therapeutic effects of fresh air and sun, and her regimen turned into fun when she brought out the lawnchairs, wrapped us in blankets, and read us her favorite tales by Hans Christian Andersen.

When my younger brother came down with severe whooping cough, Mother's loving care and treatment helped save his life, a fact admitted by our family doctor who never did hesitate to recommend old-time remedies that worked.

RECUPERATING QUICKLY WITH TASTY, NUTRITIOUS HERBAL JUICES

The value of fresh herbal juices can hardly be overestimated, for they are rich in nutrients and other healing substances. Did you know, for instance, that ½-cup of kale contains 10,000 I.U. of vitamin A, and that the juice from garden cress (*Lepidium sativum*) and garlic (*Allium sativum*) contains antibiotic substances? While these juices may not be considered to be a gourmet's delight, they are potent natural medicines. Mix these juices with other, more tasty, fruit or vegetable juices, decorate them with slices of lemon or lime, garnish with parsley or lemon balm, and you have created an attractive and potent healing drink.

Drink herbal juices immediately after extraction, or else important nutrients will be lost. If you must keep them, refrigerate in tightly covered container and add vitamin C powder (ascorbic acid) as a natural preservative.

Don't throw away the pulp. Put it in a saucepan, cover with water, and simmer for 30 minutes. Cool, strain, and store in refrigerator or freezer. Use for soup stocks and sauces.

The following herbal juices are recommended for their therapeutic effects, and only the most useful are included here. These natural medicines have been clinically tested and should be taken in small doses. Adults take one tablespoon 3–4 times daily before meals. Children take one teaspoon 3–4 times daily or less. There are no known side effects with these herbal juices.

• Artichoke (*Cynara scolymus*)—flower heads, leaves, roots. Helps arteriosclerosis; stimulates liver and gallbladder activity; helps fatigue, indigestion.

• Beans, green (*Phaseolus vulgaris*)—young leaves, young pods. Helps kidney ailments, metabolic disturbances, skin problems, diabetes, hypoglycemia. (Young green bean pods are rich in salicic acid and hormonal substances closely related to insulin.)

• Beet, red (*Ssp. cruenta*)—tops, bulb. Helps anemia, liver ailments, infections.

• Birch (*Betula alba*)—leaves. Relieves bladder and kidney ailments, arthritic diseases (diuretic).

• Borage (*Borago officinalis*). Reduces nervous tension and hysteria due to hormonal disturbances, fever.

• Cabbage, white (*Brassica oleracea*)—leaves. Aids intestinal disorders, peptic, duodenal and jejunal ulcers.

• Carrot (*Daucus carota sativa*)—root. Relieves night blindness, eye strain, infections, skin disorders.

• Celery (*Apium graveolens*)—root, leaves, seed. Aids kidney and bladder ailments (diuretic, blood cleanser), arthritic diseases, gout, flatulence, chronic pulmonary catarrh, lack of appetite.

• Coltsfoot (*Tussilago farfara*)—leaves, flowers. Relieves all respiratory disorders, asthma, bronchitis, coughs.

• Dandelion (*Taraxacum officinalis*)—root, young leaves. Helps intestinal disorders, bladder and kidney ailments (diuretic), liver ailments, faulty metabolism.

• Garden cress (*Lepidium sativum*)—leaves. Helps infections, fever, whooping cough (antibiotic, antispasmodic).

• Garlic (*Allium sativum*)—bulb. Helps arteriosclerosis, infections (antibiotic), fever, digestive disorders, flatulence, intestinal worms.

• Hawthorn (*Crataegus oxyacantha*)—flowers, fruit. Aids high blood pressure, metabolic disturbances, heart ailments, inflammation of heart muscle, arteriosclerosis, nervous heart disorders.

• Lance-leaf plantain (*Plantago lanceolata*)—plants. Relieves coughs, bronchial catarrh, tonsillitis, diarrhea.

• Nettle (*Urtica dioica*)—young leaves only. Helps arthritic ailments, bladder infections, hemorrhoids, digestive disorders. Do not overuse!

• Parsley (*Petroselinum sativum*)—whole plant, seeds. Helps arteriosclerosis, digestive disorders (blood cleanser), headaches, dizziness, fatigue.

• Radish, black (*Raphanus sativus n.*)—root. Aids liver ailments; improves gallbladder function; helps digestive disorders, spastic colon, skin disorders, arthritic diseases, coughs.

• Silverweed (*Potentilla anserina*)—herb. Relieves spastic conditions, difficult and painful menstruation.

• St. Johnswort (*Hypericum perforatum*)—plant. Good for all nervous disorders.

• Valerian (*Valeriana officinalis*)—rootstock. Aids nervous tension, headaches, insomnia, spastic conditions, intestinal cramps.

• Yarrow (*Achillea millefolium*)—plant. Helps digestive disorders, bloating, flatulence, gallbladder and liver problems (stimulates bile secretion), hemorrhage, varicose veins, nervous heart conditions, fast pulse, dizziness, headaches due to high blood pressure, hot flushes, hormonal disturbances.

****

References:

Bircher-Benner. *Bircher-Benner Nutrition Plan for Raw Foods and Juices.* Nash Publ., 1972.

Cecil-Loeb. *Textbook of Medicine.* Philadelphia, London, Toronto: Saunders, 1971.

Clark, Linda. *Handbook of Natural Remedies for Common Ailments.* Old Greenwich, Conn.: Devin-Adair Co., 1976.

Freise, Ed, Prof.; Von Morgenstern, F., Dr. *Der Drogist, Lehr- und Nachschlage buch fuer Drogisten und Apotheker.* Nordhausen: H. Killinger Verlag (no date).

Goerz, Heinz. *Gesundheit durch Heilkraeuter.* Wiesbaden: W. Moeller Verlag, 1974.

Graedon, Joe. *The People's Pharmacy.* Avon Books, 1976.

Guyton, Arthur C., M.D. *Textbook of Medical Physiology.* Philadelphia, London, Toronto: Saunders, 1971.

Lindt, Inge. *Naturheilkunde.* Koeln: Buch und Zeit Verlag, 1977.

Lust, John, M.D.,D.B.M. *The Herb Book.* B. Lust Publ., 1974.

Mendelsohn, Robert S., M.D. *Male Practice.* Chicago: Contemporary Books, 1981.

Rettenmaier, Rissmann, Ziegler, Drs. *Botanik-Drogenkunde.* Koeln: R. Mueller Verlag, 1975.

Robinson, Corinne H. *Normal and Therapeutic Nutrition.* Macmillan, 1972.

Schauenberg, P.; Paris, F. *Heilpflanzen.* Muenchen, Bern, Wien: BLV Verlag, 1978.

Sportelli, Louis, D.C. *Introduction to Chiropractic.* Sportelli Publ., 1978.

Stage, Wolfgang, M.D. *Das Kneipp Taschenbuch.* Ullstein Verlag, 1968.

"What a Headache." *Current Health.* Sept. 1978, pp. 3–10.

2

Ancient, Inexpensive Home Treatments Bring Quick Relief to Digestive Disorders

EATING HABITS CAN CAUSE OR ELIMINATE DIGESTIVE DISTRESS

An old German adage that was long ignored or laughed at says, "You are as good as your digestion." Nutritionists and modern medical researchers are now beginning to recognize the importance of proper digestion. The fact is, our modern low-roughage diet is an important cause of serious disorders, including digestive ailments. Cancer of the colon, diverticulitis, and hemorrhoids are directly related to the digestion and metabolism of food and the operation of the digestive system.

Prior to the 1880s, digestive disorders were ailments of aristocrats because only wealthy people could afford to eat white breads and other refined grains. Peasants and poor city-dwellers had to settle for "black" bread, which was made from coarsely-milled grains.

The discovery of the steel rolling mill changed all this. Precisely polished steel surfaces enabled millers to produce finer flours at low cost. Since insects are attracted to nutritious foods, such as freshly-milled flour, nutrients were soon removed to increase storage time. To attract buyers even more, fiber, which was thought to be worthless to human health, was also removed from grains. Common people were now able to eat what only royalty had consumed before: prestigious white flour.

It should be remembered that at that time the average European consumed about one pound of flour per day, mostly in the form of bread. In comparison, today's people eat about six ounces of flour per day.

One pound of this unrefined flour supplied plenty of nutrients, including vitamin E from wheat germ, plus good amounts of fiber. Since the body's capacity to digest these so-called insoluble carbohydrates is practically nil, fibers were quickly disregarded and considered unnecessary for human health. We now know, however, that dietary fiber is just as important to our health as the well-recognized proteins, fats, and carbohydrates.

In fact, researchers compiled available data and found that prior to the 1880s, appendicitis, which we accept as a common ailment, was very rare. When diets became more and more fiber-free, the incidence of appendicitis gradually became more commonplace.

Diverticular disease of the colon only emerged as a common disease after the late 1920s. Dr. David Reuben, M.D., and author of *The Save Your Life Diet*, cites statistics indicating that in Britain between 1931 and 1971 the death rate from that condition increased 600 percent.

Medical research demonstrates that the aforementioned diseases, including obesity, are virtually unknown among individuals and cultures consuming a high-roughage diet. When people like the Japanese (whose diets traditionally supply much bulk) switch to an all-American low-roughage diet, they gradually, but relentlessly, succumb to these and other digestive disorders.

Statistics indicate that this increase in digestive disorders has increased in all Western societies and is directly correlated to dietary fiber intake. In Germany an estimated 50% of all people experience digestive disorders, and serious problems such as colon cancer are on the rise. Similar studies are available for other "civilized" nations.

Food-induced ailments can be avoided—if people are willing to return to healthier eating habits. After all, so-called "primitive" civilizations that live on fiber-rich diets are nearly free of digestive disorders.

Fiber is important. It stimulates digestion by improving peristaltic movement. Unfortunately, many people are not aware that a lack of fiber causes a lazy colon which consequently results in:

1. flatulence, because starches and sugars ferment;

2. diverticulitis or diverticulosis, because large amounts of fecal material push against the intestine and produce little sacs or pouches which fill with waste material producing an ideal environment for putrefaction;

3. hemorrhoids and varicose veins may develop (or get worse), because large amounts of material collected in the intestinal tract exert pressure on the pelvic veins, creating back pressure which balloons the veins in the hemorrhoidal plexus and in the legs.

High-fiber foods assure proper digestion and are much more filling than refined products. If you are concerned about your calorie intake, that should make you think. Wholesome, fiber-rich foods will help you cut down on calories and promote proper digestion. Grains, fresh fruits, and vegetables supply plenty of fiber plus good amounts of vitamins, minerals, and certain enzymes. Fresh papayas, pineapples, and mangos are excellent digestive aids that are rich in carbohydrate-digesting enzymes. Indians, Italians, Hawaiians, and people of other cultures have long valued these foods. Try them and you, too, may say goodbye to digestive ailments.

Eating habits are often the cause of digestive problems. I vividly remember dinnertime at my grandparents' house. Eating was a ceremony with certain rituals that were all carried out in a relaxed atmosphere. TVs didn't exist yet, and nobody was allowed to read at the table, or, God forbid, grab a bite and run. People enjoyed food by eating slowly. Today's table crimes were either nonexistent or prohibited. It may sound strict, but enforcing good eating habits does promote health.

Rule 1: Chew Slowly

Digestion starts in the mouth where the enzyme ptyalin is secreted. Careful chewing stimulates the secretion of this starch-digesting enzyme which is found in the mouth only. Eat fast, and you shortchange your digestive process.

If you are a dieter trying to control eating by chewing gum, you are fooling yourself. Chewing signals to the body that food is to come, and the process of digestion starts. As a result, your stomach and pancreas get ready by producing enzymes. If, however, food is not supplied, hunger pains appear and you will crave food even more.

Rule 2: Avoid Hot and Cold Foods

Mixing hot and cold is another frequently committed modern sin. Ever since ice-makers became standard household items, people started insulting their stomachs. Your mouth, throat, and stomach are neither equipped to handle ice-cold drinks, nor do they prefer steaming-hot soups. Room-temperature drinks and foods may not seem thrilling to you, but your digestive tract does favor them.

Rule 3: Avoid Hot Spices

The excessive use of hot spices can irritate mucous membranes and actually cause ulcers. If you are prone to digestive disorders, beware.

Rule 4: Eat Small Meals Frequently

Unless you are a compulsive eater, forget about the time and eat when your body tells you to. In the old days, people ate several small, wholesome meals throughout the day, generally 2–3 hours apart, and wouldn't you know, diabetes and hypoglycemia were relatively rare. Contrary to popular belief, snackers are not obese people. I am a snacker and I have never experienced a weight problem. Eating small meals does not lead to overeating. Instead, it frequently leads to a reduction in calorie intake which translates into weight loss. Snacking helps prevent digestive problems—unless you gorge yourself with junk foods.

Rule 5: Avoid Stimulants

Did your grandparents drink coffee regularly? Mine didn't. Instead, they drank "acorn coffee," which really is a healthy herbal brew with a flavor that resembles the taste of coffee. It was not until the late 1950s, when Germany was swept by the American coffee craze, that Grandma served real coffee—and then on Sundays only.

Stimulants such as nicotine and alcohol contribute equally to digestive disorders and inhibit healing of ulcers. Both of my grandfathers smoked an occasional cigar and drank their daily single glass of beer or wine, but that was the extent of it. Neither one indulged beyond that. Analyze the eating and drinking habits of centenarians and you will notice that moderation is their key to longevity.

Rule 6: Don't Take Antacids—Unless Your Nutritionally-Oriented Doctor Tells You To

Listen to your body and you will learn which foods upset your digestion. Avoid them. It's simpler and cheaper than drug care. Unfortunately, modern pharmacology has made great advances in producing medicines that seem beneficial. Antacids fall into this category. While they temporarily and quickly eliminate stomach distress, they are capable of creating worse problems than an occasional upset stomach. Certainly, antacids neutralize stomach acidity, but what most people don't know is that antacids also stimulate the stomach's mucous membranes to produce even more acid, and when this happens, you pop another antacid, and fizz, fizz, the acid is quickly neutralized. No matter how much antacid you pour down, your stomach won't agree with a neutral, or God forbid, alkaline environment; hence, it energetically pours out more acid to create the proper acidic environment. Your stomach has to maintain a certain pH, or enzymes such as pepsin are unable to perform their jobs.

So what happens after the stomach's mucous membranes worked hard to provide plenty of acid? You get another, worse case of heartburn. You pop more antacids, you feel temporarily relieved before another heartburn returns and so on and so forth. Unless you stop and seek more natural remedies, you will continue marching down this path until ulcers make you stop. As the great German surgeon Carl Ludwig Schleich (1859-1922) once said, "We are proud of our mind, but each stomach cell is smarter than each and every studied chemist ..."

In some cases, a simple antacid such as baking soda is needed to balance the pH of the intestine, which should be alkaline. If the intestinal environment is not alkaline enough, proteolytic enzymes are unable to perform their jobs and digestion remains incomplete.

To be specific, the pH of the stomach ideally lies between 1.8 and 2.0, whereas the pH of the small intestine should be no lower than 6.8 and no higher than 9.0. The digestive system of people who are suffering from allergies and/or diabetes tends to be more acidic, and in these cases, administration of small amounts of baking soda after eating helps to correct intestinal pH.

Rule 7: Learn to Cope with Stress

If tension or stress is part of your gastrointestinal problem, you need to increase your stress tolerance. You can learn relaxation techniques by joining Yoga classes and the like; you may receive valuable feedback through biofeedback; or, you may want to read existing literature and come up with your own relaxation techniques. Sitting in a hot tub could do the trick for you, or you may prefer sitting in a cozy room, staring at the wall, listening to music, whatever. There is no technique that suits everybody, and by the same token, anything that reduces your stress level should be considered a valuable relaxation technique.

Nutritional supplements, such as high-potency B-complex vitamins, often improve stress tolerance. Since certain B-vitamins are also co-enzymes that help metabolize food, these nutrients actually support your nervous system and your digestive system as well.

But remember, while stress may be a cause of digestive disorders, most, if not all, digestive problems are food-related. If, for instance, you are popping Brewer's yeast tablets by the dozen each day and your symptoms get worse, suspect a food intolerance. It may very well be that you are allergic to the yeast. Should that be the case, any B-complex derived from Brewer's yeast would cause you troubles. Since hypoallergenic products are available now, you could switch, for example, to a rice-based B-complex. Or, if you are among those who cannot tolerate yeast or rice, try a truly synthetic brand. Although I am generally not for synthetic products of any kind, I admit that in some instances their use is justified.

Rule 8: Eat Wholesome Foods

If you already suffer from digestive problems, eat sparingly and eat the most wholesome foods available. Don't believe outdated medical advice that a bland diet will cure your problems. It does not. Supply your diet with whole grains and plenty of fresh fruits and vegetables. Always choose food that is in its most natural state. Avoid products that never spoil, because their food value is low no matter how attractive their appearance. Although chemistry can preserve foods for eternity, it cannot successfully duplicate nature. Foods loaded with additives can fool your eyes and palate, but they won't fool your body forever.

Rule 9: Don't Overeat Anything

Overeating of any food, no matter how wholesome, can create food sensitivities. If, for instance, you enjoy eating bananas, eating them every day for the rest of your life may not be in your best interest. People susceptible to any kind of allergy should be especially careful because research indicates that these individuals acquire food sensitivities easily.

Rotate your foods. Try to eat something different every day and don't come back to the same food for three to four days. This way, your system has a chance to regularly free itself of any foodstuff and won't become overly sensitized to anything.

Rule 10: Try Natural Remedies First

Most likely, your digestive problems will clear up sooner than expected and you won't have to worry about dangerous side effects. Natural remedies are safer than drugs and are often just as effective.

KNEIPP'S CENTURY-OLD REMEDY THAT STIMULATES DIGESTION

Dry-skin brushing has been popular with Europeans for centuries and was one of Sebastian Kneipp's favorite therapies for sluggish digestion. This simple, inexpensive treatment is still part of German, French, and other European health-spa treatments and while it sounds incredible, it really does stimulate circulation and digestion. Don't dismiss it before you've tried it.

Use a dry bristle massage brush, a loofah sponge, or a dry wash cloth and gently rub your abdominal area in a circular motion starting from right to left. This old-fashioned home treatment helps relieve gas and discomfort.

THE CAYCE APPROACH TO STOMACH ULCERS

Edgar Cayce, America's famous psychic healer, was enthusiastic about raw almonds and recommended their use for various ailments. In one of his many readings he stated:

"And if an almond is taken each day and kept up, you'll never have accumulations of tumors or such conditions through the body. An almond a day is much more in accord with keeping the doctor away, especially certain types of doctors, than apples."[1]

According to Dr. Harold J. Reilly, Cayce specialist, the Cayce Clinic in Phoenix is trying to launch a nationwide project that would prove the therapeutic benefits of raw almonds, which, incidentally, were endorsed by the renowned Swiss doctor, Max Bircher-Benner, over a century ago.

In addition to almonds, Cayce specifically recommended grapes in the treatment of ulcers. Grape therapies have long enjoyed popularity in European countries and continue to be endorsed by physicians of the famous Tyrolean spa, Meran, where grape cures are praised as the ideal cleansing diet.

Cayce's grape therapy for ulcers is simple:

"... And live practically on grapes during that period—or grapes and milk—with a little curd or crackers in same. The Concord grapes are preferable to be eaten ..."[2]

Incidentally, in Meran, blue grapes are also preferred and I suppose it's because of their iron content.

Cayce recommended that this type of treatment be continued for at least three to four days, and Dr. Reilly reports that in a number of patients "there was significant shrinking of tumors."

How Simon T. Treated His Peptic Ulcers

Simon T. had never heard of vitamin U, which is found chiefly in raw cabbage leaves and has been shown to have potent anti-ulcer properties.

[1]From *The Edgar Cayce Handbook for Health Through Drugless Therapy*, by Harold J. Reilly and Ruth Hagy Brod (Copyright © 1975 by Harold J. Reilly). Used by permission of Macmillan Publishing Company.
[2]*Ibid.*

What he knew, however, was that fresh cabbage juice healed his frequently recurring peptic ulcers unlike other remedies, and no doctor could persuade him to take anything else.

Simon T. seemed to be a typical ulcer patient. A perfectionist and easily irritable, he tried to conceal his feelings "like a real man." He couldn't take it easy and whenever situations got out of hand, he developed stomach distress and ultimately, ulcers.

His magic potion? One cup of fresh cabbage juice before each meal.

Since he had learned to eat several small meals a day, this meant 5–6 cups of fresh, white cabbage juice daily.

Does this century-old folk remedy work? While the discovery of vitamin U (the substance found in cabbage juice) began in the 1940s, recent research conducted by Garnett Cheney, M.D. of Stanford, indicates that it does. Ninety-two patients in whom ulcer craters could be demonstrated through X-rays were tested. Each patient was taken off any anti-ulcer medication and given cooked foods only, plus an additional one quart of fresh, raw cabbage juice divided into four or five doses per day. Eighty-six of the patients were pain-free within two weeks, and 81% of all patients were symptom-free within one week. In addition to the quick relief, X-rays demonstrated healing of the ulcers in almost every case.

You can't stand that much cabbage juice? Modify this old-time remedy by substituting part of the cabbage juice with one cup of celery juice daily, divided into five small doses, and mix the remaining cabbage juice with tomato, pineapple, or carrot juice.

FRESHEN YOUR BREATH—NATURALLY

Bad breath, like acne, won't kill you but it sure can ruin your love life. While digestive disorders are often the underlying cause of halitosis (another term for bad breath), chewing dill seeds or chlorophyll/thymol tablets as sold in health food stores can quickly freshen the worst breath and temporarily eliminate the problem. Chew one or two tablets after you eat strong foods, or heaven forbid, drink or smoke, and your mouth will feel as clean as a spring breeze.

The following old-time herbal breath freshener tea improves digestive problems, which may be the true cause of halitosis. In addition to taking the above mentioned chlorophyll/thymol tablets and chewing dill seeds, drink 2–3 cups of this brew throughout the day and soon you won't hear any complaints about your breath.

Herbal Breath Freshener Tea

1 oz. anise
1 oz. camomile
1 oz. peppermint leaves
1 oz. lemon balm
½ oz. European angelica root
½ oz. echinacea
½ oz. cloves
½ oz. parsley

Add 1 teaspoon of herbal mixture to 1 cup cold water and soak for 1 hour. Bring to boil, remove from heat, and strain after 5 minutes.

Take Susie C., who suffered from a severe case of halitosis which was relieved only temporarily by strong mouthwashes as advertised on TV. After years of agony, she started this old-time herbal program and within a week her problem disappeared, much to her great happiness.

AN OLD-FASHIONED DOCTOR'S SIMPLE APPROACH TO REDUCING STOMACH ACIDITY

The following old-fashioned recommendations are from our family doctor who, above all, enforced the following simple regimen. Try it. You will be helped like the many others before.

1. Cut fat and meat intake to a minimum as these foods stimulate acid secretion.

2. Supply diet with plenty of homemade, creamy vegetable soups to soothe mucous membranes. Creamy potato soup was our doctor's favorite medical "prescription."

3. Drink plenty of water, especially before meals. This helps to dilute stomach acidity.

4. Drink one cup of camomile tea (*Matricaria chamomilla*) with each meal. Camomile's active ingredient, azulene, effectively reduces inflammation of mucous membranes.

5. Avoid stressful situations. Anger, frustrations, and other negative feelings can cause gastric disturbances that may lead to ulcers.

6. Don't take aspirin. Vienna researchers have substantiated that acetylsalicylic acid, aspirin's main component, can be detrimental to the stomach's mucous membranes. Results indicated that 50 to 70% of all patients tested showed mucous membrane damage after aspirin use.

THE BIRCHER-BENNER APPROACH TO GASTRITIS

Chronic gastritis can be a symptom of serious illness, says Mme. Ruth Kunz-Bircher, daughter of the legendary Dr. Max Bircher-Benner of Zurich, Switzerland. Where the main cause of gastritis is bad eating habits, the Bircher-Benner treatment brings quick relief. Needless to say, the success of this dietary approach has long been established.

If you suffer from flatulence drink at least two pints of fluids daily. In any case, gastritic sufferers should have a daily fluid intake of at least one quart.

Drink at least one pint of bilberry leaf tea (*Vaccinium myrtillus*) or blackberry leaf tea (*Rubus villosus*) a day.

Eat whole-grain cereals (wheat, oat or rye) made from 2 teaspoons of cereal that has been soaked in 3 tablespoons of water for 12 hours. Cook over low heat for 10 minutes and serve.

Drink rice or barley water. Cook 1 teaspoon of grain in 7 ounces of water for 5 minutes, stirring constantly. Strain and drink. If this doesn't sound too appetizing, mix 1 part of grain water with 2 parts of fruit or vegetable juice and drink.

To soothe inflammation, drink an herbal tea mixture of approximately equal amounts of camomile (*Matricaria chamomilla*), linseed (*Linum usitatissimum*), rosehip (*Rosa spp.*), and marshmallow root (*Althaea officinalis*).

During the acute stages, your only solid foods should be cereals made from oats, linseed, or whole wheat—of which you may take 2–5 bowls daily. You may add fresh fruits and raw vegetables after recovery, but don't include oranges and grapefruits until all heartburn has stopped. Mix all juices, especially at first, with 1 part of linseed or sesame gruel.

Drink non-sparkling water only.

Dairy products: 2 or 3 yogurts per day, plus 5–6 ounces of whey or fresh buttermilk.

Drink almond milk made from 1 teaspoon almond puree mixed with ¾ water and 5–10 drops of lemon juice. No sugar or other sweeteners should be added.

For a quick recovery, eat nothing else but the foods and drinks outlined here. If you are in pain, drink camomile tea and put hot packs on your stomach. These old-time remedies will reduce discomfort and promote recovery.

If you are traveling eat three or four almonds daily but chew them slowly and thoroughly.[3]

[3]From *The Bircher-Benner Health Guide*, by Ruth Kunz-Bircher. Used by permission of Woodbridge Press Publishing Company, P.O. Box 6189, Santa Barbara, CA 93111.

CONTROLLING INDIGESTION, THE TRADITIONAL WAY

Peppermint tea (*Mentha piperita*) is one of the true old-time reme-dies for indigestion. It has been a favorite of people of nearly all cultures and continues to enjoy popularity as a tasty, healing herb. It saved me from lots of agony during the early stages of my pregnancies when indi-gestion seemed unbearable.

Peppermint tea efficiently reduces stomach distress, improves diges-tion, and relieves nausea without endangering the unborn child's life. I do recommend peppermint tea to all indigestion-sufferers and especially to pregnant women. Peppermint tea is an ideal alternative to drug treat-ment and has long been valued by German and other European health care providers.

Just recently, Dr. John Rhodes, gastroenterologist of the University of Wales, indicated that peppermint oil can relieve and soothe stomach distress. (German pharmacological research had indicated this long ago.) According to Dr. Rhodes, 13 of 16 people with intestinal distress re-ported feeling "much better" after taking a capsule of peppermint oil. Peppermint oil, the herb's active ingredient, relaxes stomach muscles and relieves abdominal pain. It also helps to dislodge air from the stomach because it relaxes the muscles at the lower end of the esophagus, thus helping you to burp.

Martin Furlenmaier, M.D., a noted Swiss authority on phyto-therapy (= herbalism), homeopathy, and chiropractic, indicated that the therapeutic effects of peppermint oil are beneficial in the treat-ment of indigestion, but, Dr. Furlenmaier added, peppermint's other ingredients are equally beneficial. Like many of his European colleagues, he believes that it may be more beneficial to use the whole herb rather than isolated compounds.

According to Dr. Furlenmaier and others, peppermint is an effec-tive antispasmodic that has calming and antiseptic properties and is particularly useful in the treatment of colics and spastic conditions. European studies indicate that peppermint oil stimulates gallbladder se-cretion ninefold! Hence, it should *not* be taken by people suffering from heartburn. The herb also reduces tension headaches.

RELIEVING STOMACH PAIN WITH ACUTHERAPY

Stomach pain? Test the side of your knee, just below the knee cap, for tender spots. Most likely, you will notice an area that is extremely sensitive to the touch. Massage it until most of the local pain disappears, and correspondingly, the stomach discomfort you experienced will diminish.

I used this old-time Chinese remedy during the early stages of my last pregnancy when stomach pains and nausea caused considerable discomfort. I found great relief from this simple home treatment. I have since recommended it to a number of patients, most of whom noticed temporary improvement.

NEW AND OLD WAYS TO CONTROL COLIC

Indigestion, improper foods, or constipation may be the cause of colic. Nutritional research shows that a potassium deficiency causes the contraction of intestinal muscles, which slows down markedly or results in partial or complete paralysis of these muscles. Potassium deficiency occurs after severe diarrhea, surgery, or other forms of stress and may be the result of a poor diet that is high in refined foods and salt. Certain drugs such as cortisone and diuretics are also known to induce potassium deficiency. A study of 655 colicky infants revealed that the lower the potassium level, the worse the colics became.

In most cases, potassium levels can be restored by eating a diet that supplies liberal amounts of fresh fruits and vegetables. Potassium deficiency-related colics generally disappear quickly after an adequate diet.

In Germany and other European countries, colics are treated with a warm infusion of fennel tea (*Foeniculum vulgare*). This simple, old-time home remedy brings quick results and is safe for people of all ages. Colicky infants quickly respond to this popular European treatment which mildly relaxes and promotes digestion.

Valerian root (*Valeriana off.*) is an excellent antispasmodic for severe and persisting colic. In Germany, this well-established medicinal herb is used for a variety of ailments, including menstrual cramps, nervous headaches, insomnia, diarrhea, and colic due to nervousness. Germany's famous medical doctor Hufeland called valerian root the best "medicine" for nervous disorders, hysteria, and colics, and prescribed this herb in small doses to many of his patients with good results. Valerian should not be taken over long periods of time as this may cause headaches and nausea in some individuals.

The following modified herbal formulas have long been endorsed by Austrian, German and Swiss doctors to treat flatulence and colicky conditions. Use 1 teaspoon of herbal mixture per 1 cup boiling-hot water. Strain after 3–5 minutes and drink 1 cup after meals and before bedtime.

Herbal Tea Formulas for Colic

Formula 1

1 part celandine (*Chelidonium majus*)
1 part valerian (*Valeriana off.*)
2 parts European centaury (*Erythraea centaurium*)
5 parts caraway (*Carum carvi*)

Formula 2

1 part sweet flag (*Acorus calamus*)
1 part fennel seed (*Foeniculum vulgare*)
2 parts valerian (*Valeriana off.*)
3 parts German camomile (*Matricaria chamomilla*)
3 parts peppermint (*Mentha piperita*)

Formula 3

1 part ginger (*Zingiber officinale*)
1 part thyme (*Thymus vulgaris*)
1 part valerian (*Valeriana off.*)
2 parts peppermint (*Mentha pip.*)
3 parts camomile (*Matricaria chamomilla*)

A hot foot bath or a hot pack placed over the abdominal area relaxes and provides relief to colicky patients.

PROVEN EUROPEAN HERBAL TEA MIXTURES THAT STRENGTHEN YOUR STOMACH

European Stomach Strengthener

Formula 1

1 oz. gentian root (*Gentiana lutea*)
1 oz. wild clover (*Trifolium pratense*)
1 oz. European centaury (*Erythraea centaurium*)
1 oz. ground fennel seed (*Foeniculum vulgare*)
1 oz. ground horehound (*Marrubium vulgare*)

Formula 2

1 oz. German camomile (*Matricaria chamomilla*)
2 oz. fennel seeds (*Foeniculum vulgare*)
2 oz. European centaury (*Erythraea centaurium*)

Formula 3

Useful for ulcer-prone individuals. Use equal parts of:

gentian root (*Gentiana lutea*)

angelica root (*Angelica sylvestris or A. atropurporea*)
St. Johnswort (*Hypericum perforatum*)
sweet flag (*Acorus calamus*)
camomile (*Matricaria chamomilla*)
peppermint (*Mentha piperita*)
European centaury (*Erythraea centaurium*)
wormwood (*Artemisia absinthium*)

Formula 4

Soothing and healing to entire gastrointestinal tract, including liver and gallbladder.

2 oz. yarrow (*Achillea millefolium*)
2 oz. fennel seeds (*Foeniculum vulgare*)
2 oz. European centaury (*Erythraea centaury*)
1 oz. dandelion root (*Taraxacum officinale*)
1 oz. licorice root (*Glycyrrhiza glabra*)
1 oz. German camomile (*Matricaria chamomilla*)
1 oz. valerian root (*Valeriana officinalis*)
½ oz. lemon balm (*Melissa officinalis*)
½ oz. caraway seeds (*Carum carvi*)

We have used this stomach strengthener in a more specific combination in our practice with great results. Patients who have suffered from digestive distress for years found quick relief after using this herbal tea.

Preparation of above formulas:

Use 1 teaspoon per 1 cup cold water. Bring to boil, remove from heat, and steep for 3–5 minutes. Strain and drink 1 cup with each meal.

European Bitter Tonic 1

2 oz. gentian root (*Gentiana lutea*)
2 oz. wormwood (*Artemisia absinthium*)
½ oz. Valerian root (*Valeriana officinalis*)
Soak 1 teaspoon herbal mixture in 1 cup cold water for 8–12 hours, bring to quick boil, strain and drink in mouthful doses.

Remember that the healing herbal formulas outlined here are not meant to please your palate. If they do, so much the better. These teas are natural medicines that have been used by European folk healers for centuries and continue to be endorsed by modern health care providers. Visit an Austrian, German, or any other European drugstore and you will find similar medicinal herbal formulas displayed and advertised.

SIMPLE HOME TREATMENTS FOR COLITIS

Inflammation of the large bowel, or colon, is referred to as colitis, a condition that accounts for 50 to 70% of all gastrointestinal complaints. Causes include excessive use of laxatives or cathartics, antibiotic therapy, food allergy, poor diet, chronic constipation, and emotional upsets. Nervous individuals who have difficulties coping with stressful situations are especially prone to colitis.

Pain due to gas or vigorous contractions of the colon is the most frequent symptom of colitis. Such pain may be dull, sharp, or intermittent and is sometimes accompanied by lack of appetite, nausea, vomiting, even headaches and heartburns. Stools are usually dry and hard and may contain large amounts of mucus. In severe cases, ulcers form and cause bleeding and hemorrhage.

Adelle Davis and other noted nutritionists reported that colitis patients are often severely deficient in vitamins A, C, E, all the B-vitamins, potassium, magnesium, fat, protein, and practically all nutrients. We found in our practice that a highly nutritious diet supplemented with the above vitamins and minerals quickly improves patients' conditions. In addition, one cup of camomile tea (*Matricaria chamomilla*) or marshmallow root (*Althaea officinalis*) taken before meals quickly reduces inflammation and relieves discomfort.

GYPSY REMEDIES AND OTHER ANCIENT TREATMENTS THAT OVERCOME CONSTIPATION

Mrs. Maria, descendant of an old Hungarian gypsy dynasty, believed that constipation is the enemy of every health-conscious individual. Her remedy was simple: "Chew one handful of linseeds (*Linum usitatissimum*) during the day, or eat linseed bread."

The recipe for this delicious, fiber-rich bread is simple: substitute one cup of flour with one cup of linseeds, also referred to as flax. Linseeds are rich in fatty acids, pectin, mucilaginous content, and roughage and are excellent for people who experience too much gas after eating bran. Linseeds are tasty, tend to reduce inflammation, and stimulate bowel movement. Discover linseeds and you won't ever need laxatives again.

We all know the importance of roughage. Bran certainly helps to stimulate peristaltic movement, yet foods such as beets contain plenty of roughage, too, plus good amounts of vitamins and minerals (especially iron). If you suffer from constipation, try eating one or two small beets and you will have a good bowel movement about 12 hours later. Instead of constipating iron supplements, I often recommend beets to anemic patients suffering from constipation, and this old-fashioned remedy quickly eliminates digestive problems and does wonders for liver ailments and anemia. Beets are wonderful foods. They are on my menu at least once a week.

My grandmother, like many Europeans, believed that one glass of water taken before breakfast helps regulate bowel movement. Prune juice is recommended when problems are more persistent.

Jethro Kloss, author of *Back to Eden,* recommended deep breathing exercises "... and in the morning before getting up, lie on your back, knees flexed, and pant, breathing in short, rapid gasps. Roll on your side, face, and left side, and continue panting." It sounds strange, yet it works. This exercise does massage and stimulate the bowels.

Chiropractic adjustments work similarly. Many of our patients who come in for low back pain, soon notice that bowel movements become more regular. Helen R. called it "a nice and unexpected benefit."

If you are looking for a harmless herbal laxative, try the following German formulas that have been used for generations.

Mild Herbal Laxative

2 parts marshmallow root (*Althaea officinalis*)
2 parts licorice root (*Glycyrrhiza glabra*)
3 parts sassafras (*Rhamnus frangula*)
3 parts rhubarb (*Rheum palmatum*)

Use 1 teaspoon herbal mixture per 1 cup cold water. Bring to quick boil, reduce from heat, and soak for 1 hour. Drink 1 cup mornings or evenings.

Potent Herbal Laxative

1 part fennel seeds (*Foeniculum vulgare*)
2 parts senna leaves (*Casia acutifolia*)
2 parts sassafras (*Rhamnus frangula*)

Use 1 teaspoon herbal tea mixture per 1 cup cold water. Let soak overnight, strain, and drink 1 cup in the mornings. Longer steeping or heating up will increase strength and possibly cause cramping.

INEXPENSIVE KNEIPP REMEDIES FOR HEMORRHOIDS

Hemorrhoids are often treated like an embarrassing joke, but they are nothing to laugh about. They are merely varicose veins in an awkward place. Hemorrhoids are often caused by constipation and may be painful whether they are internal or external. Occasional bleeding may bring some relief.

Sebastian Kneipp's famous water treatments have withstood the test of time and numerous European doctors incorporated his regimen. Kneipp Clinics, as well as the Bircher-Benner Sanatorium, prescribe cold sitz baths in addition to exercise and a wholesome, fiber-rich diet, free of all hot spices, coffee, and alcohol.

Sitz baths are simple. Fill your tub halfway with water. If you want to speed up the healing process, add one gallon of cold camomile infusion (*Matricaria chamomilla*) to the tub water. Bath temperature should be between 15 and 20 degrees Celsius (= 60 to 70 degrees Fahrenheit). Slowly immerse your lower body into the water and remain there for a few minutes. Get out quickly, dry yourself, apply zinc ointment to external hemorrhoids, take a zinc supplement, hop into bed and rest.

We have recommended this old-fashioned therapy to many of our patients with excellent results.

MY PARENTS' SECRET HOME REMEDY THAT QUICKLY STOPS DIARRHEA

Instead of drugs, we used to sell refined charcoal tablets to customers who needed quick relief from diarrhea, and this old-fashioned remedy always worked.

During my father's imprisonment in Russian camps, many of his comrades came down with cholera, a condition that claimed the lives of thousands of prisoners in Russia and elsewhere. Father was able to save many people, and his treatment was simple. He burned certain plant roots and fed this coal to the ailing. Recovery seemed miraculous, though there was no miracle involved. Coal acts as a filter, cleansing the intestines of putrefactive bacteria.

Of course, it would be foolish for you to eat burned roots. Instead, use Mother's modified remedy that is even simpler. Necessary requisites are a toaster and sliced bread. Slightly burn the bread. In severe cases, toast bread repeatedly and eat. You should be free of diarrhea within a short time. To speed up recovery, drink one or two cups of camomile tea.

I recommended this simple home treatment to a special friend in distress. After all else had failed, this natural therapy quickly put her back on her feet. Needless to say, this old-time folk remedy has proven useful many times.

ASIAN AND EUROPEAN FOLK TREATMENTS THAT CONTROL AND PREVENT INTESTINAL BACTERIA

Itching around the anus may be a sign of intestinal parasites, yet you don't need to panic. Treatment is easy. Try this old herbal therapy which has been used by American and South American Indians, as well as most Asian cultures, and which eventually found its way into European herbalism. This inexpensive folk remedy is highly effective and I find it surprising how unknown it is among American health care providers. But then, selling pumpkin seeds is not promising business ...

Yes, pumpkin seeds (*Cucurbita pepo*) are safe and powerful anthelmintics that help expel or destroy intestinal worms, especially tapeworms. Chew a few roasted pumpkin seeds per day for prevention, and a handful or more to expel intestinal parasites.

To speed up recovery, drink a cup of carrot juice per day. Carrot juice is another potent anthelmintic that can safely be given to people of all ages, particularly infants. This sweet-tasting juice contains essential oils that effectively expel roundworms, prevent putrefaction in the intestine, help gastrointestinal catarrh, and reduce stomach acidity and heartburn. Carrot juice is high in potassium, hence it acts as a mild and natural diuretic.

In case you like neither one of the above old-time remedies, make use of another ancient herbal treatment that Semitic priests used centuries ago. Today, thyme (*Thymus vulgare*) is listed in nearly all European pharmacopoeias. Drink one cup of thyme tea per day or take two to three drops of thyme oil on a sugar cube two or three times daily. Thyme oil, the plant's chief constituent, is an effective antiseptic and parasiticide which effectively expels hookworms.

Garlic is another useful anthelmintic that continues to enjoy popularity among all cultures. It helps all intestinal problems including infections. Cold-pressed garlic oil has been successfully employed in the treatment of pinworms and in fact, intestinal parasites are seldom found among garlic lovers.

HOW THE BULGARIANS PREVENT DIGESTIVE DISORDERS

The longevity of the Bulgarian people is legendary and their health secrets are simple:

1. They eat a wholesome and unadulterated diet that includes plenty of fermented foods such as kefir and yogurt made from goat milk.
2. Food is eaten sparingly.
3. Indulging is a luxury reserved for other cultures.
4. Hard, physical work is part of the Bulgarians' daily lives.

Americans may consider themselves one of the most fortunate and healthiest of people, yet disease and mortality rates indicate otherwise. Certainly, the majority of Americans find the Bulgarians' meager lifestyle unappealing, yet health benefits are obvious. A long, healthy life should be worth sacrifices. If health and longevity is what you want, you had better evaluate and possibly change your present lifestyle.

Start out by avoiding junk food that is loaded with chemical additives. Each day, statistics keep pouring in, indicating that a wide range of ailments such as allergies, digestive disorders, hypertension, and even cancer are related to food additives. Preservatives, colorings, and flavorings can all be linked to disease and should be avoided as if they were poison, which they are.

Eat foods that are in their most natural state and stay away from fast foods. If you don't always have time to cook old-fashioned, wholesome meals, feast on yogurt, whole grains, and fresh fruits and vegetables. If you use your imagination, you may come up with fantastic meals that do not require heating up a single food, which will save you plenty of time for recreation—and most of all such raw foods provide valuable vitamins, minerals, and enzymes.

Stay away from drugs. If you need health care give natural remedies a first try. It will save you lots of trouble.

Exercise and be merry, and you will have plenty of reasons to look forward to a fruitful, healthy, and long life.

****

References:

Baker, Charles E., Jr. *Physicians' Desk Reference*, 35th edition. Medical Economics, 1981.

Cecil-Loeb. *Textbook of Medicine.* Saunders, 1971.

Colimore, Benjamin, M.A.; Colimore, Sarah Stewart, L.P.T. *Nutrition and Your Body.* Light Wave Press, 1974.

Davis, Adelle. *Let's Get Well.* Harcourt, Brace and World, Inc., 1965.

Donsbach, Kurt, Ph.D. *Nutrition in Action.* Int. Inst. of Natural Health Sciences, Inc., 1977.

Fredericks, Carlton, Dr. *New and Complete Nutrition Handbook.* Int. Inst. of Natural Health Sciences, Inc., 1976.

Freise, Ed., Prof.; Von Morgenstern F., Dr. *Der Drogist.* Killinger.

Furlenmaier, M., M.D. *Wunderwelt der Heilpflanzen.* Rheingauer Verl., 1978.

Goerz, Heinz. *Gesundheit durch Heilkraeuter.* W. Moeller, Verl., 1974.

Graedon, Joe. *The People's Pharmacy.* Avon Books, 1976.

Guyton, Arthur C., M.D. *Textbook of Medical Physiology.* Saunders, 1971.

Harvey; Bordley. *Differential Diagnosis.* Saunders, 1970.

Heinermann, John. *Science of Herbal Medicine.* By-World, 1979.

Kloss, Jethro. *Back to Eden.* Woodbridge Press, 1972.

Kunz-Bircher, Ruth. *The Bircher-Benner Health Guide.* Woodbridge, 1980.

Lindt, Inge. *Naturheilkunde*, Buch & Zeit Verl., 1977.

Lust, John, N.D. *The Herb Book.* Lust Publ., 1974.

Mendelsohn, Robert S., M.D. *Confessions of a Medical Heretic.* Contemporary Books, 1979.

Morscher, Betsy. *Heal Yourself the European Way.* Parker, 1980.

Pfeiffer, Carl C., Ph.D., M.D. *Mental and Elemental Nutrients.* Keats, 1975.

Reilly, Harold. *The Edgar Cayce Handbook for Health through Drugless Therapy.* Macmillan, 1971.

Rettenmaier; Rissmann; Ziegler, Ph.D.s. *Botanik-Drogenkunde.* R. Mueller Verlag, 1975.

Reuben, David, M.D. *The Save Your Life Diet.* Random House, 1975.

Robinson, Corinne H. *Normal and Therapeutic Nutrition.* Macmillan, 1972.

Selye, Hans, Ph.D. *Stress Without Distress.* Signet Books, 1974.

Spoerke, David G. Jr. *Herbal Medications.* Woodbridge Press Publ., 1980.

Stage, Wolfgang, M.D. *Das Kneipp Taschenbuch.* Ullstein, 1978.

Verrett, Jacqueline; Carper, Jean. *Eating May Be Hazardous To Your Health.* Anchor Books, 1978.

Williams, Roger J., Ph.D. *The Wonderful World Within You.* Bantam, 1977.

Muetter Magazin, 6, 1978, p. 4.

Der Wegweiser, Der Bote aus der Aotheke, 1979, 5, p. 8.

———— .   1979, 16, p. 3.

———— .   1979, 24, p. 2.

———— .   1981, 4, p. 21.

———— .   1981, 3, p. 15.

———— .   1981, 9, p. 17.

Reform Rundschau, 1979, 9, p. 10.

———— .   1979, 11, p. 9.

———— .   1980, 6, p. 33.

———— .   1980, 8, p. 8.

———— .   1981, 1, p. 20.

———— .   1981, 4, p. 16.

3

Helping Arthritis
and Other Chronic Diseases,
the Old-Fashioned Way

SOME FACTS ABOUT ARTHRITIS

Nearly 35 million Americans suffer from arthritis and related diseases, and despite modern medicine's advancements, this major crippler is more common than ever. The incidence of arthritis is rapidly increasing in persons of all ages, and many arthritics, for whom pain is a fact of daily life, have taken refuge in painkillers and other drugs. As a result, drug abuse is common among arthritis sufferers.

Arthritis is a puzzling disease, and the various forms of this potential crippler have different causes and symptoms. Thus, what helps one individual does not necessarily benefit the other.

Understandably, arthritis victims are not encouraged by these prospects. But in order to find a helpful therapy it is imperative to know with what form of arthritis the individual is afflicted, and what might have caused or contributed to the disease.

Psychiatric theory claims that arthritis is a psychologically-induced disorder, while biochemical or nutritional researchers define it as a metabolic stress disease, and recent medical research indicates that the disease may be hereditary or a manifestation of an impaired immune system. Most likely, arthritis is a combination of all of the above and should be approached as such.

Presently, rheumatologists recognize about 100 different types of arthritis with the most common forms being rheumatoid arthritis, osteoarthritis, and gout.

Rheumatoid arthritis is an extremely common form which affects several joints simultaneously and is typified by chronic joint inflammation that often affects the small joints of the hand. It is the most crippling of the three types of arthritis and generally starts between the ages of 20 and 45. It affects three times as many women as men, and in severe cases inflammation and thickening of tissue around joints causes destruction of bones, deformity, and eventually disability. While its true cause is unknown, some researchers believe the disease may be sparked by a virus. Nutritionists and biochemists think rheumatoid arthritis is linked to a disruption of the body's immune system.

Osteoarthritis, also called the "wear-and-tear" disease, is a form of degenerative disease. Chronic irritation of the joints, often found in overweight individuals and those with poor posture, a previous injury, or occupational strain all contribute to the onset of osteoarthritis. Older people, particularly women, are the most frequent victims and this may indicate a hormonal involvement such as reduced estrogen production. More than 70% of Americans over the age of 55 are afflicted with osteoarthritis.

Gout is the easiest form of arthritis to diagnose and treat. It certainly is the best understood of all arthritic ailments. Nearly all cases of gout occur in men. Gout is the result of a uric acid imbalance which causes joint inflammation and usually affects one joint at a time. It generally starts when too much uric acid is deposited in the tissues and attacks may follow minor injury, excessive eating or drinking, overexercise, or surgery. In some cases, attacks occur for no apparent reason and are severely disabling. Thought to be hereditary, gout often afflicts the joints in the foot and knee.

Other forms of arthritis include *juvenile arthritis* which primarily affects those under 16 years of age and causes growth disturbances. The disease, which is similar to the form that afflicts adults, can produce high fever and skin rash and statistics suggest it to be more common than ever.

Less common forms are:

Allergic arthritis, which is caused by allergies.

Gonorrheal arthritis, which is the result of severe gonorrhea.

Hemophilic arthritis, the result of a hemophiliac's bleeding, causes stiffening and inflammation of joints.

Tuberculous arthritis is the result of an infection with tuberculosis appearing as secondary infection.

Psoriatic arthritis affects about 10% of the people suffering from psoriasis, a common and sometimes severe skin disease. Psoriatic arthritis afflicts more women than men, most of whom are between 20 and 40 years of age.

Rheumatoid spondylitis affects mostly young males. Its main symptoms are back pain, stiffness, and loss of spinal mobility.

No matter what type of arthritis an individual is afflicted with, a sound diet, moderate exercise, and staying in control of emotional ups and downs can do much to improve well-being. After all, everything we do and don't do affects us physically as well as psychologically. How we cope with stress, what we eat, and how our body is tuned determines our state of health.

There are no shortcuts. Health is each individual's responsibility, and if lost, no doctor will be able to restore it all by himself. Living the natural way is far simpler than surgery and certainly preferable to drug therapy.

Old-fashioned arthritic remedies provide one avenue to better health. If used wisely, they successfully relieve the aches and pains arthritic sufferers are so familiar with, enabling individuals to be active and enjoy life to its fullest.

ANCIENT ARTHRITIC REMEDIES FROM AROUND THE WORLD

The disease of arthritis dates back to antiquity. Bones of the Java ape man and the mummies of Egypt show signs of arthritic damage, as do skeletons of prehistoric dinosaurs.

Arthritis afflicts people of all economic backgrounds, races, and nationalities, and over the centuries folk healers developed special herbal remedies aimed at reducing suffering. Some of these ancient antidotes withstood the test of time.

In the Balkans folk healers make a special rosmarin liquor that is used like today's alcoholic medicines. This remedy is made from three cups of vodka and one cup of rosmarin leaves (*Rosmarinus officinalis*) which are both added to a large bottle. After being tightly corked, the content is shaken three times daily and left in the sun or near a hot stove for three days. The liquor is then strained into another bottle and after a pinch of camphor (*Cinnamomum camphora*) is added, this alcoholic remedy is rubbed into painful joints or muscles which are then covered with warm cloths. The arthritis sufferer also takes eight drops of this liquor internally one to three times daily, depending on the severity of the case and until pain eases.

This old-fashioned remedy has a fine taste the Russians have enjoyed for centuries. My father, while a prisoner of war, saw it used among Russian guards and he once actually persuaded a guard to share some of his remedy which was then used to ease a comrade's aches and pains.

Long before the war my father had prepared a similar medicine after a pharmaceutical recipe dating back 60 years or more. Today, Spiritus Rosmarini, as modern druggists call the remedy now prepared from rosmarin leaves and ethanol, is still included in German pharmaceutical text books, and rosmarin leaves, known for their anti-inflammatory action, are listed in the German pharmacopoeia.

Spiritus Rosmarini is still sold in German drugstores. In some cases, it is sold as Dr. X's Rheumatoid Ointment, or is simply labeled:

Spiritus Rosmarini

Ointment for rheumatism and arthritis
External use: gently rub onto affected area.
Internal use: ½ tsp. three times daily with water.

The Japanese used to treat arthritic symptoms with a hot bath and a traditional cup of warm basil tea. These remedies were equally popular among the people of India long before medicine recognized the benefits of hydrotherapy, and before it was established that basil (*Ocimum basilicum*) strengthens the kidneys and bladder and is an antispasmodic that has the ability to reduce pain.

The American Indians preferred drinking a mixture of mashed yucca root in water, one of the oldest Indian arthritic remedies, and its effect has been explained by modern scientists.

Yucca saponin, a steroid derivative of the yucca plant, is a precursor to cortisone, the hormone which was once highly publicized as a treatment for arthritic ailments. However, yucca saponin does not produce the side effects associated with cortisone therapy, and a double-blind study done at a Southern California arthritis clinic demonstrated the healing power of yucca, which Indians knew about for centuries.

During this study yucca in tablet form was administered to 165 patients ranging in age from 11 to 92, and neither doctor nor patient knew whether the "medicine" given was yucca or a placebo. Sixty percent of all patients receiving yucca showed dramatic improvement of arthritic problems and among the beneficial "side effects" were relief from headaches and improvement of gastrointestinal disorders.

HOW THE EUROPEANS APPROACH ARTHRITIS

When the Europeans "discovered" fancy milling and refining procedures a number of diseases, arthritis among them, started to rise to an all-time high. Many of these ailments have been on the increase ever since. Just recently, Professor H. Warning, M.D., of Saarbrücken, West

Germany, pointed out new statistics which suggest that 30% of all West Germans are afflicted with arthritis which costs the West German government an estimated 18 to 20 billion German marks per year. Now, government officials are trying in vain to reduce costs in a world of rising prices. Since recent statistics indicate that drugs are not highly successful in the treatment of arthritic diseases, more attention is focused on natural therapies.

Natural arthritic liniments containing herbs such as wintergreen, witch hazel, and willow bark are making a comeback, and for good reasons. Willow bark products, for instance, contain salicin, a bitter, white, crystalline glycoside believed to be converted to salicylic acid in the body. Salicylic acid is known for its anti-rheumatic properties, and is closely related to aspirin.

For more than two thousand years, willow bark hot packs and salves have helped arthritis sufferers. Willow bark (*Salix alba*) relieves pain and inflammation, is a good diuretic, and has no known side effects.

Willow bark salve is easy to make. Add crushed bark or powdered bark into a small pot, add sufficient olive oil or peanut oil to cover, and simmer for about one hour. Strain through paper filter and cool. Use as a pain-soothing rub.

To make a *willow bark hot pack* use 3 teaspoons of powdered herb, moisten with enough hot water to make a paste, and apply to affected area. Wrap dry cloth around and leave until cold. Wash area and cleanse with camomile tea (*Matricaria chamomilla*).

Willow bark tea helps to eliminate toxins and waste fluids and strengthens the system. Make a tea by soaking 2 teaspoons dried, crushed bark in 1 cup cold water and bring to quick boil. Remove from heat, strain after 5 to 10 minutes, and drink one cup a day in small doses.

While abroad, I ran into Mrs. H. who, years ago, had helped my mother with household chores. More of a friend than a maid, she helped wherever needed and we children enjoyed her because she could stand an awful lot of noise—except when pain troubled her arthritic knees.

Those were the times when mother applied the usual willow bark hot pack and brewed her "rheumatism tea." I remember those incidents because the next day Mrs. H. always showed up with her delicious apple strudel and worked as hard as ever.

It is impossible to talk about arthritic remedies without mentioning the great German healer Sebastian Kneipp, whose remedies are now manufactured and distributed by Europe's largest pharmaceutical company, and whose followers include chiropractors, medical doctors, naturopaths, and osteopaths.

To aid aching joints and to stimulate circulation Kneipp often "prescribed" rosmarin baths, and today Kneipp's rosmarin bath is as appreciated by arthritic victims as much as it was nearly 100 years ago. German, Austrian, and Swiss drugstores carry Kneipp's products, and my mother swears that a rosmarin bath takes care of most minor aches and pains.

To make such a bath add one handful of rosmarin leaves to one pint of cold water. Bring to a quick boil, remove from heat and let soak for one hour or more. Strain liquid and pour into tub water. The remaining leaves can be used to strengthen tub water by putting them into a linen bag which can be hung into the tub for additional extraction.

Dr. Wolfgang Stage of Bad Wörishofen has practiced Kneipp methods since 1963. According to him, oat straw is particularly beneficial to those arthritic victims suffering from nervousness and insomnia. Dr. Stage recommends vinegar-and-oat straw packs for local pain, and oat straw baths to improve patients' general well-being.

Vinegar-and-Oat Straw Pack

To make a vinegar-and-oat straw pack, add 1 part vinegar to 3 parts oat straw infusion (boil ½ pound of oat straw in 1 qt. water for 30 minutes). Wet towel, wring out excess fluid, and apply to affected area. Repeat when needed.

An oat straw bath is made by adding 3 qts. of oat straw infusion to the tub water.

In addition, Kneipp health spas emphasize exercise, particularly "water wading," which is nothing more than walking in cold water. Some health spas make use of rivers, others have their patients wade in small basins. Generally, 10 to 20 minutes of wading are encouraged, and this simple treatment, Kneipp doctors insist, is known to stimulate arthritic sufferers' often faulty metabolisms. Studies indicate that this simple but well-known Kneipp therapy has caused amazing improvements in arthritic patients.

ANOTHER OLD-FASHIONED HERBAL REMEDY FOR ARTHRITIC PAIN

Father was fond of herbal packs and his knowledge of medicinal herbs—their properties and uses—convinced many skeptics. One of our town's general practitioners never thought much about herbal remedies but after drug treatments failed to help his osteoarthritis he reluctantly tried father's remedies. He applied an herbal pack containing angelica root (*Angelica archangelica*) and birch leaves (*Betula alba*) whenever pain troubled him, and drank his daily cup of birch leaf tea in the morning and another one or two cups of father's special angelica-birch leaf-comfrey mixture during the day. After a few weeks the good doctor admitted to feeling better.

Why? Angelica root is a good tonic and mild diuretic; comfrey improves gastrointestinal function; and birch leaves prevent calcium loss.

Professor H. Wagner, Director of the Pharmaceutical Institute of the University of Munich, recently substantiated the old claim that birch leaves are highly beneficial to arthritic ailments.

The Norwegians and Laplanders have made use of birch leaves for ages, and one of their herbal remedies is unlike all others.

Nordic arthritics bury themselves in a bed of fresh birch leaves, leaving only their heads uncovered. They then try to relax, which isn't easy, because soon an itching sensation is felt that is followed by an outburst of sweating. After that, they say, the pain eases and they feel fresh and full of energy.

Unusual as it may seem, this treatment is far less exotic than the ones European farmers recommend. "Sit in a stinging nettle bed," they tell arthritic sufferers, or "lie on an ant hill," though the advice is usually given with a smile.

HOW THE ROMANS EASED ARTHRITIC PAIN

During my last trip to Germany, I came across an eye-catching article about a "Roman spa" that had been used over 2,000 years ago by Roman soldiers troubled with the aches and pains of arthritis. In 1979, these ancient healing springs were reopened to serve modern man.

This Roman spa, located in the village of Birnbach, a quiet rural community in the foothills of Southeast Bavaria, has existed since 3,000 B.C., and the springs are, indeed, effective in treating arthritic and rheumatic ailments. Modern balneologists (balneology is the science of the therapeutic use of baths) from the Institute of Balneology and Climatology, and the Chemical Balneological Institute of the Technical University of Munich have officially declared that the high mineral content in combination with the springs' high temperatures are of therapeutic value to all arthritic diseases. As a result, hydrotherapy and adjunct treatments at the spa are covered by Germany's national health insurance.

The springs are known as the Sodiumhydrogencarbonate-Chloride Thermae. As the name implies, spring water is high in sodium, hydrogencarbonate, and chloride and contains good amounts of potassium, magnesium, calcium, manganese, iodine, iron, sulfur, and silica, plus free carbon dioxide.

Indoor and outdoor pools range in temperature from 28° to 38° (=82°-100°F) Centigrade. Patients soak or perform special exercises in these baths, receive underwater massage, and are encouraged to relax in the solarium.

Hydrotherapists indicate that the natural organic substances and inorganic matter present in the water influence the body's physiological and chemical reactions. Endocrine function is stimulated which is important for the arthritic patient. Adrenal function, it is known, is often critical among arthritis sufferers.

While at the spa I met Walter S. of Munich, who had been troubled with chronic rheumatoid arthritis for years. Painkillers had caused additional problems and cortisone injections, though helpful at first, had changed him into a "junkie," he said. When he finally realized that there was no improvement in sight he changed physicians. His new doctor slowly took him off drugs and sent him to this Roman spa where a whole new approach was started. After 3½ weeks of continuous treatments, Walter S. felt better than he had in years. Underwater therapy, massage, a better diet, programmed exercise, and rest changed Walter S.'s life for the better.

HOW SPINAL MANIPULATION HELPS RELIEVE ARTHRITIC MISERY

During the February 1980 conference of the AMA Orthopedic Council, Dr. Ronald Lawrence, M.D. gave the following definition of manipulation:

"Manipulative therapy involves the application of accurately determined and specifically directed manual forces to the body. The object is to improve mobility in areas that are restricted, whether the restrictions are within joints, connective tissues, or in skeletal muscles. The consequences may be the improvement of posture and locomotion, and the relief of pain and discomfort; the improvement of function elsewhere in the body; and the enhancement of the sense of well-being."

Human tissue manipulation was described in the ancient Chinese book, Kong Fou, which was written about 5,000 years ago. In ancient India physicians relieved pain by methods similar to those used by today's chiropractors and osteopaths and reported marvelous results. The ancient Egyptians believed that men and women are stronger when their spine is in perfect form and symmetry, and Herodicus, a contemporary of Hip-pocrates, achieved fame by curing diseases through spinal manipulation.

Today, many people afflicted with rheumatoid arthritis have found relief through spinal manipulation. Stiffness slowly disappears as does pain and discomfort.

A year ago I was asked to write an article about Spears Chiropractic Hospital, America's only licensed nonmedical hospital known for its natural approach to disease, particularly chronic arthritis.

Located in Denver, Colorado, Spears Hospital has been in opera-tion since 1933. Now operated by the second and third generation of Spears doctors, it continues to aid chronic sufferers from all over the country.

While visiting, I met an outspoken Southern lady who had been referred to the hospital by friends.

"Before I came here," Mrs. R. said, "my rheumatoid arthritis had become progressively worse and I constantly felt sorry for myself. I didn't want all those pills and I was scared of surgery. I knew I needed to lose weight and my diet wasn't the best. But if you can't move, you can't cook; and if you feel down, it's pretty hard to convince yourself to diet. I live alone and life just didn't look good any more."

Mrs. R. finally convinced herself that she needed intensive care. She came to Spears where she received spinal manipulation, sometimes twice daily, physical therapy, hydrotherapy, and massage. She learned to exer-cise stiff joints, and started a weight-reduction program. After five weeks of controlled health care Mrs. R. felt better than she had in years. She certainly did not feel lost and helpless any more.

At Spears, success stories are easy to come by, and I asked Dr. Raymond Spears what he can do that other chiropractors or osteopaths cannot, and whether patients recover faster if hospitalized at Spears.

"Chiropractic hospitalization," he said, "is beneficial to certain people. There are those who are disabled and need around-the-clock care; others have to have their environment changed in order to im-prove; and a lot of times it is difficult for a patient to jump in the car, ride a number of miles to the doctor's office, get the treatment and jump in the car again, and go home and wait for two days for another treatment. This is where chiropractic hospitalization comes in."

RELIEVING PAIN WITH CHINESE REMEDIES

Nobody in his right mind enjoys pain, and over the centuries, people have found ways to escape suffering. Some Indian yogis use meditation; some Persians habitually smoke opium; and while many Western people made generous use of painkilling drugs, many Orientals instead use acupuncture or acupressure to block pain-carrying nerve impulses.

Acupuncture or acupressure, more precisely defined as Meridian therapy, has been successfully applied for thousands of years. Historians say ancient warriors wounded by spears and arrows, or weavers accidentally punctured by needles often recovered from certain diseases, a phenomenon also observed in tortured criminals.

Wise men of ancient times tried to unveil this mystery through experimentation. They pierced skin, first with bamboo sticks and later with bronze needles, and found it was possible to duplicate certain effects. Specific points on the skin corresponded with particular ailments, a connection discovered over 5,000 years ago. Since these points for curing disease do not follow along nerve lines, Western doctors and scientists have difficulties understanding the concept.

Acupuncture, commonly associated with the use and insertion of needles, received its name from Jesuit missionaries traveling through China during the seventeenth century. Acupuncture is clearly a Western translation. "Acus" stands for needle; "pungo" for puncture.

Acupressure, the application of finger pressure to the points, has not received much attention yet, though it requires much less knowledge and skill and can actually be practiced by the patient.

Pressure points are easy to locate. They are areas which are tender and sensitive to pressure. Applying pressure first causes local pain which slowly decreases until the pressure point is pain-free. When this happens, corresponding problems such as hip pain, stomach problems, or a toothache may disappear even though the pressure point is often located in a seemingly unrelated part of the body. In some instances, however, acupressure points are at or near the center of pain.

Arthritic pain may be controlled by acupressure (see figures that follow). Mr. G. came to our clinic because he was afflicted with arthritic knees and was frequently tortured by sudden attacks that rendered him helpless. My husband taught the man to massage the corresponding acupressure points (see knee pain figure on page 66) and since all points were extremely tender, Mr. G. had no difficulty locating each one. He massaged all points as instructed, and in general, his pain eased. This saved him lots of trips to the office. Needless to say, this quiet senior citizen is very fond of Meridan therapy.

See the following figures which illustrate the particular acupressure points that ease different areas of arthritic pain.

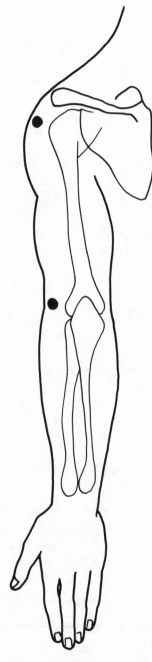

General Acupressure Points for Rheumatoid Arthritis

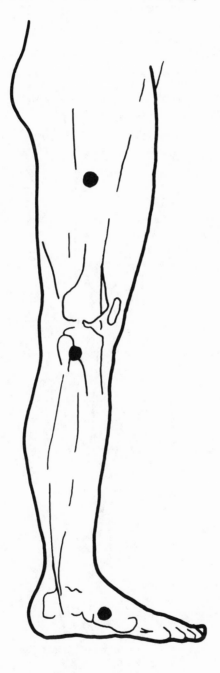

Acupressure Points for Hip Pain

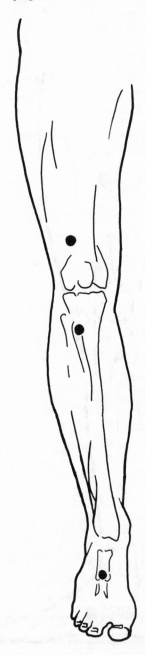

Acupressure Points for Knee Pain

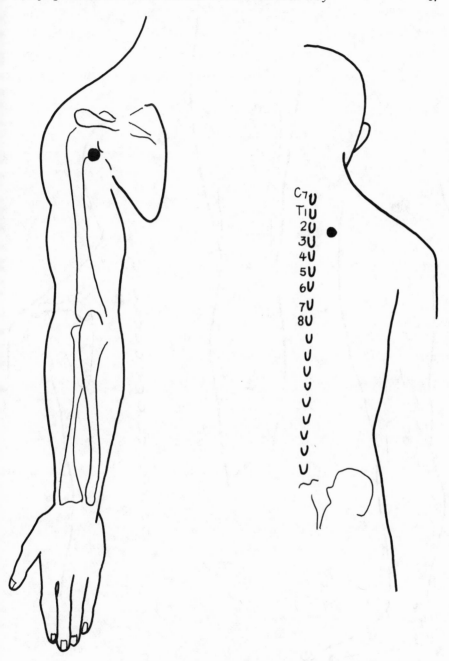

Acupressure Points for Shoulder Pain

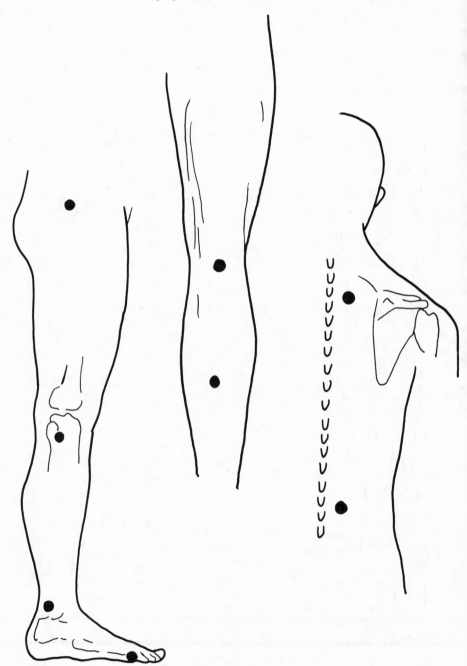

Acupressure Points for Sciatica

AN OLD-FASHIONED DIET FOR GOUT

Gout has been called the "sickness of the kings" for it prevails in well-to-do societies where eating rich foods and drinking wine is customary. Though said to be hereditary, gout usually disappears at wartime when food is scarce and people largely rely on unrefined grains, fruits, and vegetables.

Generally speaking, anybody suffering from gout should eat several small meals consisting of wholesome food and fruit juices, especially cherry and citrus juices which help to keep uric-acid crystals in solution and stimulate their excretion. Drinking three quarts of liquid per day is recommended, and herbal teas such as sarsaparilla, milfoil (yarrow), rosehip, and peppermint aid the condition. Other foods such as sauerkraut and radishes are helpful because they improve digestion and are rich in sulfur, the mineral most arthritic patients are deficient in.

A "raw food diet" is used at the famous Bircher-Benner Clinic of Zurich, Switzerland, known for its natural approach to health care. This simple dietary program has brought great relief to thousands of gout victims.

Recommended Foods

Fresh and lightly cooked vegetables, particularly celery, which is a mild diuretic. Liberal amounts of fresh fruits should be eaten daily. Sugar-free yogurts and cottage cheese supply protein as do eggs, which are also rich in sulfur. Whole grain breads and cereals should replace all refined baked goods, but need to be excluded from the diet during attacks.

Forbidden Foods

Red meats, salt, strong spices such as pepper, curry, and paprika, caffeine, soft drinks, all sweets, refined foods, and alcohol.

A recent FDA report indicates that two professors at Rutgers University theorized that vegetables classified as "nightshades" might cause arthritic conditions. Among these vegetables are tomatoes, white potatoes, green peppers, and eggplant. Though further evidence is needed, all arthritic sufferers—gout victims included—should carefully evaluate whether symptoms correspond with certain dietary habits and eliminate foods that prove to be detrimental. It is my opinion that arthritis patients often suffer from food and chemical allergies, and while nightshades affect some patients, there may be additional involvements. A food sensitivity test could reveal surprising facts.

How Ellen M. Dealt with Bursitis

At age 23, Ellen M. suffered from bursitis, a chronic inflammation of the bursa, a small sac containing fluid that lies between a tendon and the bone over which the tendon moves. "Tennis elbow" or "housemaid knee" are folksy names describing the areas that this painful and debilitating disease most commonly affects.

In Ellen's case both shoulders troubled her immensely, and this highly-skilled secretary was often unable to perform simple chores. When she came to our office seeking an alternative to drug therapy, she was close to losing her job.

Ultrasound, a high-frequency vibration treatment known to penetrate living tissue, helped reduce pain almost instantly. Since ultrasound helps the body absorb calcium deposits and clear up inflammation of the bursae, it was applied during office visits and proved to be highly beneficial.

At home, Ellen M. used a hot linseed poultice to reduce pain, and always followed this self-treatment with a gentle stroking massage.

To make a pain-relieving linseed poultice use linseed powder or crushed seeds and mix with hot water until a smooth paste is formed. Apply to affected area and leave on until cold.

Ellen also loved to indulge in junk foods; a diet profile and mineral analysis showed her to be deficient in important nutrients. This convinced Ellen that a wholesome diet was necessary to improve her general well-being, and she soon ate a healthy diet that supplied her body with much-needed protein derived from milk products, eggs, fish, and some meat. Ellen was advised to eat fresh papaya fruit, which is rich in digestive enzymes, take additional digestive enzymes, and the nutritional supplements vitamin A, B-complex, C, iron, and the minerals calcium and magnesium.

Since Ellen had a tendency to tighten up her shoulders when under stress, we asked her to reduce anxieties to a minimum and learn to relax her shoulder muscles.

Under this program Ellen's condition soon improved. She was able to keep her job, and eventually advanced to a better position.

COPING WITH OSTEOPOROSIS

About 40% of those aged 65 and older are afflicted with osteoporosis, a deficiency disease characterized by a reduction of total bone mass. Though no change in the structure of chemical composition of bones occurs, bones become less dense and more fragile, and fractures occur easily. In some cases, vertebrae collapse spontaneously without causing any gross injury, with most patients actually unaware that this has happened. At times, however, pressure to the nerve roots may cause intractable pain, muscle spasms set in, and the patient suffers from severe and persistent backaches.

X-rays are presently the only reliable means of diagnosing the condition, and spinal manipulation, known to be valuable to back pain, should be administered with care and only after a thorough X-ray examination or fractures may result.

Unfortunately, roentgenographic changes are not obvious until as much as 30% of the bone mass has been lost, and osteoporosis is in an advanced state. Blood analysis generally shows normal levels of calcium, phosphorus, and proteins, though an inadequate intake of these nutrients and others such as the collagen-building vitamin C, and a defect in the synthesis of proteins is the reason osteoporosis in the spine prevails in women 45-years-old and older. Since hormonal and nutritional factors are interrelated, pregnancy and menopause are believed to accelerate the disease, unless the patient pays close attention to her nutritional deficiencies.

People suffering from osteoporosis are known to lose height, sometimes up to four inches within a single year. This phenomenon is caused by collapsing vertebrae, and in some cases leads to severe kyphosis (hump back).

Osteoporosis is among the diseases in which medicine has made no progress. A balanced diet (see "Foods and Herbs for Healthy Bones" later in this chapter), moderate exercise to prevent calcium loss, and a gentle massage to relax spastic muscles to prevent aches and pains continue to be the best and most successful therapy.

Margot T. suffered from severe osteoporosis and an examination revealed that the 67-year-old lady had compression fractures in the mid- and lower back causing muscle spasms that were responsible for excruciating pain. As a result, Mrs. T. rarely moved, which alone causes calcium to be lost from the body. Since she had a history of kidney stones, fear prevented her from eating calcium-rich foods, and Mrs. T.'s diet was nearly devoid of this much-needed mineral.

Had she known that the nutritional supplements dolomite and bonemeal, mineral combinations of calcium, magnesium, and other needed nutrients prevented stone formation, Margot T. could have avoided much suffering. Magnesium, we now know, makes calcium soluble, thus preventing calcium precipitation and vitamin D, essential to osteoporosis victims, helps to improve absorption of calcium and mineralization of bone.

Margot T. learned to improve her diet. Soft tissue manipulation relieved muscle spasms and pain and within a few weeks Mrs. T. took her first walk in a long time, a daily exercise she has enjoyed ever since.

PREVENTING BACKACHES WITH SIMPLE EXERCISES

If you complain about an aching back, you are among 75 million adults that have at least once suffered from severe and prolonged back pain. Backaches, experts say, are the second leading cause of pain in the United States, right after headaches, and according to the National Health Center for Health Statistics, another seven million sufferers are added annually.

Structurally weak, our back has to bear a great load at any time and under the worst conditions, thus making it highly susceptible to pain. Back muscles lacking strength will fail to keep the body erect, and stress or strain placed on bones and ligaments will cause problems. Overworked muscles, when under tension, react by knotting up, causing painful spasms. The result of such muscular strain is back pain.

Our muscles are as good as we make them, and a properly exercised body is able to cope with unexpected stress or strain. Alf Nachemson, the Swedish physician who designed the Volvo seat, has demonstrated that a man bending over to lift a 50-pound weight puts approximately 660 pounds of pressure at the juncture of the lumbar and the sacral spine. No wonder muscles, tendons and ligaments, if improperly exercised will go on strike, or worse, be severely injured.

Exercise is vital in strengthening back muscles, and should be done regularly and in accordance with an individual's capability. Following are a few simple exercises that will strengthen your back. Do them daily and you will soon appreciate better spinal health.

1. *Easy-to-do routine exercise.* Lie flat on back, knees bent, feet flat on floor. Use stomach and lower back muscles to lift up buttocks. Hold five seconds. Repeat. Now do reverse. Press back flat on floor allowing no space between buttocks, back and floor. To do this correctly, tighten buttocks and abdominal muscles and stay "glued" to floor. Relax. Repeat. (See Figure 1.)

2. *Leg extension to strengthen low back muscles.* Stand tall, holding on to chair and gently swing leg backwards. Do not arch. (See Figure 2.)

3. *Forward stretch.* Stand up, legs apart. Bend over and hang your arms down. Bounce gently, keeping back rounded. If you can't do this, you most likely have a back problem and need professional help. (See Figure 3.)

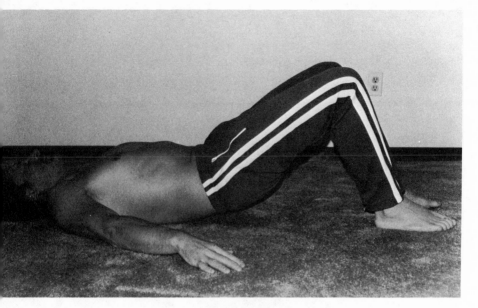

Figure 1

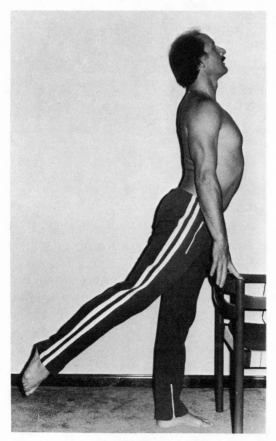

Figure 2

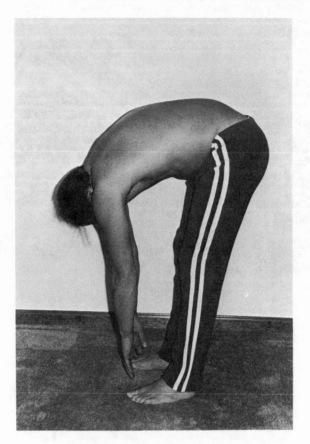

Figure 3

HELPFUL HINTS FOR SCIATICA

Sciatic pain is nothing to laugh at. If irritated or injured, the sciatic nerve, the branches of which run from the hip back down the thigh to the foot and toes, generates severe pain that is frequently provoked and aggravated by certain postures or movements, by jarring, jolting, even coughing, sneezing, or straining the stool. The pain can be so severe as to prevent the afflicted from moving; worse yet, it often makes resting and sleeping difficult.

Chiropractic manipulation generally brings great relief from pain. Acupressure (see previous section, "Relieving Pain with Chinese Remedies" in this chapter) also controls pain and soothes symptoms.

A warm poultice made from fresh horseradish root is beneficial to sciatica and other ailments affecting the peripheral nerves. According to

Dr. Martin Furlenmaier, M.D., Swiss authority on phytotherapy (another, fancier name for herbalism), such a poultice relieves nerve inflammation. Other poultices made from shave grass or linseed also relieve pain, and contrasting showers stimulate a sluggish metabolism and improve circulation.

Herbal teas such as yarrow (*Achillea millefolium*), lemon balm (*Melissa officinalis*), hops (*Humulus lupulus*), or peppermint (*Mentha piperita*) should replace all caffeinated drinks. These herbs are excellent antispasmodics that have a calming effect on the nervous system. Valerian tea (*Valeriana officinalis*) is a good sedative that relieves discomfort.

Sciatic patients usually benefit from extra vitamin C, B-complex and additional thiamine (B-1), nutrients that positively influence the nervous system. Brewer's yeast, whole grain foods, fresh fruits and vegetables should be part of the diet, unless food allergies prohibit the dietary intake of certain foods or nutrients.

> Martha S., a teacher with a history of backaches dating back 10 years, had suddenly developed severe pain along her right leg. Orthopedic surgeons confirmed sciatic problems and a disc syndrome, recommending hospitalization and surgery. Martha S. sought an alternative. We put her on the program outlined above and within two and a half months she was nearly symptom-free and able to function again. Her recovery was a victory to all involved.

CONTROLLING SCOLIOSIS

Scoliosis is the most deforming orthopedic problem confronting children, and according to Rene Cailliet, M.D., chairman and Professor of the Department of Rehabilitation Medicine of the University of Southern California's School of Medicine in Los Angeles, this once-considered rare ailment is now present in approximately two percent of the adult population.

The term scoliosis implies an abnormal curvature of the spine. Though thought to be hereditary, the true causative factors of this skeletal problem which is most acute in children is still unknown. Scoliosis is present in girls on a ratio of 9:1 as compared with boys, and if not recognized and treated in its early stages severe spinal malformation results.

To date, conventional treatment includes bed rest, traction, bracing, and in more progressive cases, surgery. Exercise is a nonsurgical procedure that has been used for centuries with good results, yet doctors often neglect to promote it.

During the seventeenth annual convention of the German Work Association for Chiropractic and Osteopathy held in Bad Kissingen, West Germany, I attended a seminar on scoliosis treatment. The lecture focused on special exercises, massage and manipulation. According to Ms. Roeb, lecturing physiotherapist, correction of scoliosis complication *is* possible through proper and continuous efforts.

A young woman 20 years of age was brought in and treatments were demonstrated. "Before" and "after" X-rays showed that the patient's severe scoliosis had improved significantly. Surgery was not discussed any more, but Ms. Roeb said, "corrective treatments had been administered daily for one and a half year."

Few people have the perseverance and stamina to go through such a strict regimen. Those who do can avoid progression of the disease. Complications such as cardio-pulmonary impairment, often seen in scoliotic patients, can be prevented. Back pain does not have to debilitate and surgery *can* be avoided.

I can testify to that. Dr. Allenberg, Clinic Director of the Northwestern Chiropractic College located in St. Paul, Minnesota, after reading my X-rays, classified me as the "best-looking, most pain-free cripple" he had ever seen. Though not entirely symptom-free, I had not been aware of the severity of my scoliosis. When I sought Dr. Allenberg's opinion I was over 30 years old and had never been to a chiropractor before. My husband, then a sophomore at the college, had arranged the visit, suspecting what no doctor had ever thought of, namely, that the occasional severe headaches and the numbness I frequently experienced in my left leg could be related to my scoliotic spine.

After two months of treatments my headaches were gone, and in the years since I have rarely experienced another one. The numbness in my leg which was once medically classified as "internal varicose veins" disappeared completely, and no one knows how grateful I am for that.

My scoliotic spine improved visibly. I still receive treatments and I exercise as much as possible. I am still very flexible and plan to stay that way.

The program is relatively simple. Manipulation plus specific exercises are aimed at (1) decreasing existing abnormal curvature of the spine, (2) reducing the thoracic (rib) hump, and (3) strengthening weak muscles to counteract curvature and hump.

Exercises are aimed at strengthening weak muscles, which generally are located opposite the scoliotic hump. There is a strong tendency among scoliosis patients to be one-sided. Muscles in the hump area are more developed, adding the clearly unwanted cosmetic effect and leading to progression of the problem. Patients also need to learn to avoid habits such as carrying weights or small objects like purses on the side that is overdeveloped. Instead of leaning into the hump, the scoliotic patient needs to straighten up his spine with the help of formerly neglected muscles. This improves lung function and generates an improved sense of well-being.

1. This touch-the-ceiling exercise is aimed at stretching muscles opposite the hump. If done correctly, a good stretch is felt all along the rib cage. Do 5 to 10 times. (See Figure 4.)

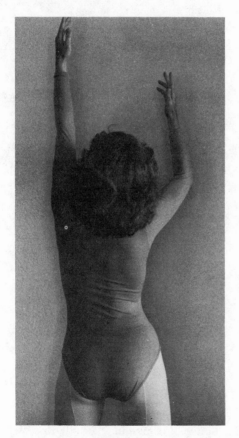

Figure 4

2. The side stretch also improves rib cage muscles. Stretch sideways as much as possible, but don't jerk and don't use shoulder joints. (See Figure 5.)

3. The side extension exercise is done only on the side opposite the hump. If done correctly, a stretch is felt in the weak muscle area. It is a strenuous exercise, and most important to the scoliotic patient. (See Figure 6.)

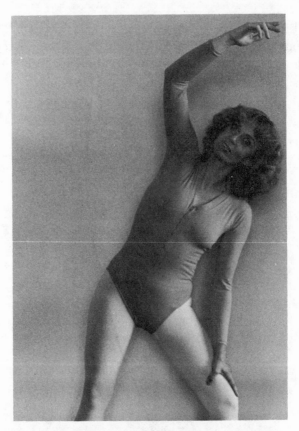

Figure 5

FOODS AND HERBS FOR HEALTHY BONES

The high incidence of osteomalacia, a disease characterized by softening of the bones in the adult which is equivalent to rickets, and osteoporosis and other arthritic diseases can be attributed to an inadequate diet. A mild fall, says Dr. Carlton Fredericks, one of America's

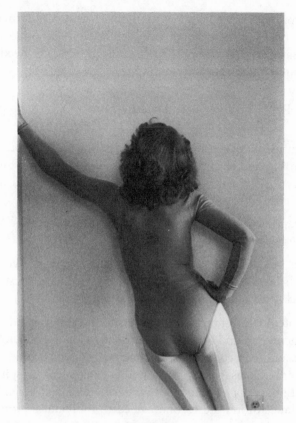

Figure 6

leading nutritionists, does not have to result in fractures. If it happens, it most likely is linked to a vitamin D, calcium, and phosphorus deficiency.

We commonly assume that when we get older we need less nutrients. Nothing could be more erroneous. Bones change constantly, and if not adequately nourished, are left brittle and weak. Bone cells die, decalcification starts, and if this development is not halted by the supply of adequate protein and any nutrient needed to utilize it, permanent damage results. Vitamin C is essential to connective-tissue formation. Dr. Roger J. Williams, nutritional pioneer, says, "When relatively large amounts of this harmless nutrient (vitamin C) are taken by mouth, the cells that produce collagen are able to appropriate it and are helped to do a better job." Dr. James Greenwood, a Houston, Texas neurosurgeon, discovered that vitamin C is useful in the treatment of neck and back pain.

Vitamin D, calcium, and phosphorus are vital to healthy bones. Dr.

Lutwak, Professor of Medicine of the University of California, believes that 1,000 mg daily of calcium completely prevents osteoporosis and related diseases. Other minerals such as magnesium are needed to balance calcium metabolism.

Basic Rules that Promote Healthy Bones

1. Get plenty of sunshine. Sunshine falling on skin converts ergosterol in and within the skin to vitamin D, the substance necessary for normal bone growth. Milk and bonemeal also supply vitamin D.

2. Exercise. Walk whenever possible to keep mobile. Immobility causes calcium loss.

3. Eat calcium-rich foods such as dairy products, whole grains, nuts, and sesame seeds. Dandelion greens, kale, mustard greens, and turnips are also good sources of calcium.

4. Protein foods such as dairy products also supply good amounts of magnesium and other vital nutrients such as sulfur. Other magnesium sources are: beans, bran, whole grains, Brussels sprouts, chard, clams, nuts, peas, prunes, raisins, and spinach. Nutritional supplements containing calcium and magnesium in a balanced form are recommended to individuals prone to stone formation.

5. Take plenty of vitamin C. Five hundred mg per day are recommended to promote production of collagen and help prevent neck and back pain. Vitamin C occurs naturally in most plants. Acerola fruit, rosehips, papaya fruit, raw green peppers, parsley, watercress, broccoli, strawberries, and other fruits are all good sources. Eat fresh fruits and vegetables whenever possible as vitamin C dissolves in water and is destroyed by prolonged cooking methods.

6. Herbal teas such as rosehips, strawberry leaves, blue violet leaves, catnip, young nettle leaves, dandelion leaves, spearmint, and raspberry leaves all supply vitamin C and other needed vitamins and minerals. Acorn tea tastes and looks much like coffee and has been recommended for centuries to promote healthy bone growth.

****

References:

Airola, Paavo O., N.D. *There IS a Cure for Arthritis.* Parker Publ. Co., 1968.

Alexander, Dale D. *Arthritis and Common Sense.* Conn: Witkower Press, 1968.

Austin, Mary, Dr. *Acupuncture Therapy.* ACI Publ., 1972.

Bircher-Benner Nutrition Plan for Arthritis and Rheumatism. Nash, 1972.

Bircher-Benner Nutrition Plan for Raw Food and Juices. Nash, 1972.

Bircher, Ralph, M.D. "Rheuma durch Vieleiweiss." *Reform Rundschau* 6, June 1980, 570th edition, p. 19.

Bircher, Ralph, M.D. "Knochenschwund durch Fleischkost." *Reform Rundschau,* Jan. 1980, 565th edition, p. 21.

Bricklin, Mark. *The Practical Encyclopedia of Natural Healing.* Rodale, 1968.

Buchheister, Ottersbach. *Handbuch der Drogistenpraxis.* Springer, 1914.

Caillet, Rene, M.D. *Scoliosis—Diagnosis and Management.* Davis Co., 1975.

Clark, Linda, M.A. *Handbook of Natural Remedies for Common Ailments.* Devin-Adair Co., 1976.

Cheraskin; Ringsdorf; Clark. *Diet and Disease.* Keats Publ., 1968.

Davis, Adelle. *Let's Get Well.* Harcourt, Brace & World, 1965.

Fidelsberger, H., M.D. "Wenn im Alter die Gelenke steif werden." *Der Bote aus der Apotheke,* Heft 18, 30. Jahrgang 1979, Sept. 1979, p. 2.

"Hocus-Pocus as Applied to Arthritis." *FDA Consumer.* Sept. 1980, p. 24.

Ford, Norman. *Secrets of Staying Young and Living Longer.* Harian, 1979.

Federicks, Carlton, Ph.D. *New and Complete Nutrition Handbook.* Major Books, 1976.

Freise, Ed; Von Morgenstern, F., Ph.D.s. *Der Drogist, Lehr- und Nachschlagebuch für Drogisten und Apotheker,* Killinger.

Furlenmaier, M., M.D. *Wunderwelt der Heilpflanzen.* Rheimgauer Verlag, 1978.

Görz, Heinz. *Gesundheit durch Heilkräuter.* Moller Verlag, 1974.

Graedon, Joe. *The People's Pharmacy.* Avon, 1976.

Grieve, M. *A Modern Herbal.* Vol. I and II. Dover, 1971.

Guyton, Arthur C., M.D. *Textbook of Medical Physiology.* Saunders, 1971.

Heinerman, John. *Science of Herbal Medicine.* By-World Publ., 1979.

Heuser; Pennell, Drs. *The "How To" Seminar of Acupuncture for Physicians.* International Pain Control Institute, 1973.

Jarvis, D.C., M.D. *Arthritis and Folk Medicine.* Holt, Rinehart and Winston, 1960.

Jenness, Martin E., D.C., Ph.D. *An Illustrated Guide to Physical Fitness.* International Health Institute, 1976.

Kester, Nancy C.; Kopell, Harvey P., M.D.s. Help for Your Aching Back. Grosset & Dunlap, 1969.

Kitay, William. New Facts About Bursitis. Crowell, 1953.

Lindt, Inge. Naturheilkunde, Heilkräuter und ihre Anwendung, Krankheiten und ihre Behandlung. Buch und Zeit Verlag Gmbh, 1977.

Lust, John, N.D., D.B.M. The Herb Book. Bantam, 1974.

Lehnert-Schroth, Ch. Grundlegende Gedanken zu den atmungs-ortho-pädischen Skoliose-Übungen nach System "Schroth". Gustav Fischer, 1976.

Potterton, David, N.D. "Rheumatoid Arthritis, Dramatic Results Through Natural Therapy." Bestways. April 1980, p. 28.

Reilly, Harold J.; Brod, Ruth Hagy. The Edgar Cayce Handbook for Health Through Drugless Therapy. Macmillan, 1975.

Reinert, Otto C., D.C., F.I.C.C. How to Live with a Bad Back. Marian Press, 1977.

Rettenmaier; Rissman; Ziegler, Ph.D.s. Botanik-Drogenkunde. R. Müller, 1975.

Robinson, Corrine H. Normal and Therapeutic Nutrition. Macmillan, 1972.

Schauenberger, Paul; Paris, Ferdinand. BLV Bestimmungsbuch, Heilpflanzen, Erkennen-Anwenden. BLV Verlag, 1978.

Selye, Hans, M.D. Stress Without Distress. Lippincott, 1974.

Smith, William Ashbury, M.D. Gout and the Gouty. Naylor, 1970.

Stage, Wolfgang, M.D. Das Kneipp Taschenbuch. Ullstein, 1968.

Spears Newsletter #178, June/July 1980, p. 1.

Williams, Roger J., Ph.D. Nutrition Against Disease. International Institute of Natural Health Sciences, Inc.

Williams, Roger J., Ph.D.; Kalita, Dwight K., Ph.D. A Physician's Handbook on Orthomolecular Medicine. Pergamon Press, 1977.

Ziegler, H. Lander A. Drogisten Praxis. München: Luitpold Lang, 1960.

4

Folk Remedies of Yore
Can Energize Your Vital Organs

IMPROVING YOUR LIFESTYLE

Your lifestyle plays a crucial role in preventing or overcoming disease, and while it is difficult to break old habits, it is not at all impossible. Quit blaming heredity or the environment for your condition and start changing the odds. It can be done. You do not have to be among the 3.9 million Americans that suffer from diabetes and related carbohydrate disorders. You can be among those who avoided or improved their condition through simple dietary changes alone.

A healthier lifestyle is in your best interest. The medical researchers, Drs. Cheraskin and Ringsdorf, Jr., point out that there is overwhelming evidence that chronic disorders generally develop over an extended period of time. "It is a fact," these scientists say, "that one does not retire well and awaken the following morning with a chronic disease. Thus, the classical identification of these problems is preceded by an incubation period, in some cases of many years' duration."

It is alarming but true. Present health care methods are not adequate to resolve even the morbidity pattern of this nation. As Drs. Cheraskin and Ringsdorf pointed out in their book, *Predictive Medicine: A Study in Strategy ... A Plan for Maintaining Health by Avoiding Disease*, Keats Publ., the United States ranks eighteenth with 24.8 deaths per 1,000 live births, and with all the billions spent for health care since 1900, the 45-year-old white male has gained only three years in life expectancy. Above this age, the increase in longevity quickly dwindles to insignificance. In other words, today's 60-year-old white male can expect to live one and one-half years longer than his grandfather did.

It is alarming, but statistics recently released by the American Heart Association indicate that 13.2 percent of Americans in the 45- to 54-year age group have heart disease, and the United States National Center for Health Statistics reveals that 27,000,000 Americans, or one out of every eight Americans, are living with some form of cardiovascular disease. Similar statistics reveal that every year approximately 55,000 people die from renal failure and 200,000 individuals develop kidney stones. Medical research also predicts that simple dietary changes would reduce acute conditions and deaths by 20%.

Each year, digestive disorders cause a loss of 8.495 million work days and 5.013 million school days. Twenty million acute conditions are reported annually and 4,000 cases are added each day. In 1976, the Census Bureau reported that according to medical studies dietary changes alone caused a 25% reduction in these disorders and cut medical costs by over one billion dollars per year.

Drs. Cheraskin and Ringsdorf, along with other medical researchers, showed overwhelming evidence that proper nutrition and changes in lifestyle can substantially reduce disease. As the researchers state, "Whether one succumbs to disease or remains unscathed is a function of the world he lives in and one's capacity to withstand external bombardment." Or, as Dr. J.M. May so eloquently phrased it, "Some people are made of glass and shatter under the slightest environmental challenge," while others appear to be structured of steel and are able to tolerate most anything.

According to statistics most of us belong to the first category, and in order to improve resistance and reduce disease susceptibility changes in lifestyle and eating habits are needed. Such changes are not easily made, and often irreversible damage has been done before people even consider making improvements.

Awhile ago, I talked with a young woman who suffers from a multitude of problems of which the main one was recurring kidney infections, but when I pointed out that a change in diet and lifestyle was needed, her reply was: "There has to be an easier way" and "Without a little fun" (by which she meant alcohol, cigarettes, coffee, and junk food) "life won't be worth a darn." Sound familiar?

I admit to have little tolerance for such ignorance and I hope you are more concerned about your health than this young lady. Take the following lifestyle quiz, and if you answer "yes" to questions 1 through 15 and "no" to questions 16 through 20, you are to be congratulated. You live a healthy lifestyle. Keep up the good work. If, however, improvements are needed, do yourself a favor and start making necessary changes *today*.

LIFESTYLE QUIZ

Part 1

1. Do you prefer herb teas, spring water, and fresh juices to alcohol, coffee, and soft drinks?   Yes   No
2. Does your diet supply enough fiber?   Yes   No
3. Are you trying to eliminate junk foods?   Yes   No
4. Do you eliminate sweets as much as possible?   Yes   No
5. Do you avoid chemical additives such as artificial colorings and flavorings and preservatives?   Yes   No
6. Do you read labels when shopping?   Yes   No
7. Do you prefer fresh foods to convenient foods?   Yes   No
8. Do you minimize your fat intake?   Yes   No
9. Do you eat well-balanced small meals, rather than one or two big meals that are high in sugar, fat, and protein?   Yes   No
10. Do you eat a wholesome breakfast?   Yes   No
11. Do you eat small dinners?   Yes   No
12. Do you consume approximately 2–3 teaspoons of polyunsaturated fats daily?   Yes   No
13. Is your cholesterol level 190 or lower, and your triglyceride level 100 or lower?   Yes   No
14. Can you tolerate stress reasonably well?   Yes   No
15. Do you exercise regularly?   Yes   No

Part 2

16. Do you frequently use aspirin or any other drug?   Yes   No
17. Do you smoke?   Yes   No
18. Do you live in a highly polluted area?   Yes   No
19. Are you overweight?   Yes   No
20. Do you go on crash diets rather than on one providing sensible weight loss?   Yes   No

GERMAN RESEARCHERS ENDORSE
HERBAL TREATMENT FOR LIVER DISEASES
INCLUDING HEPATITIS AND JAUNDICE

The liver, our largest organ and gland, is vital to a healthy, well-functioning body and is perhaps our main defense against cancer. Located under the diaphragm and above and to the right of the stomach, it activates thousands of chemical reactions, among them the production of enzymes and the regulation of the body chemistry of fat. The liver synthesizes many amino acids used in building tissues; breaks down proteins into sugar and fat; and produces lecithin, cholesterol, bile, and blood albumin which is vital to the removal of tissue wastes. It produces prothrombin which is essential to blood clotting; converts sugar into glycogen, often referred to as body starch; stores iron and several other trace minerals; destroys harmful substances such as histamine; and detoxifies potentially destructive substances such as drugs. In short, being good to your liver is like doing yourself a great favor.

An inadequately functioning or diseased liver greatly influences the body as a whole, and until recently treatment was less than satisfying. Diet and rest seemed the only avenue to recovery.

Now, German pharmacists and related health care professionals are rediscovering an old-time therapy for patients suffering from liver diseases, particularly hepatitis and jaundice.

Milk thistle (*Sylibum marianum*), one of the most beautiful thistles, is a useful medicinal herb that protects and helps to regenerate liver cells. Dr. Furlenmaier writes that milk thistle "has a specific affinity for the liver" and if used correctly is a great healer.

Milk thistle's main component is silymarin which has been found to protect liver cells from invading toxins. According to German studies, silymarin is able to counteract both lethal and sublethal poisons and give full protection for up to six hours by preventing toxins from penetrating through the cell membrane into the cell nucleus. German reports indicate that various liver diseases can be helped with old-time milk thistle preparations.

Milk thistle tea can be made by soaking 1 tsp. of milk thistle fruits in 2 cups boiling hot water for 10 to 20 minutes. Strain and drink in small doses throughout the day for prevention. Patients suffering from liver problems should drink 1 cup before each meal, and take 1 cup mixed with peppermint tea before retiring.

USEFUL FOLK REMEDIES FOR FATTY LIVER DISEASE AND CIRRHOSIS

In addition to milk thistle preparations, other old-fashioned herbal treatments aid liver problems. The following medicinal herbal tea mixtures are particularly popular natural European remedies that promote regeneration of liver cells.

Formula 1

Liver and gallbladder tea.

2 oz. milk thistle (*Sylibum marianum*)
1 oz. chicory leaves and rootstock (*Cichorium intybus*)
2 oz. dandelion root (*Taraxacum off.*)

Use: 1 tsp. per 1 cup hot water. Bring to quick boil and steep for 5–10 minutes. Drink 2–3 cups per day before meals.

Formula 2

Stimulates liver and kidney function.

1 oz. barberry (*Berberis vulgaris*)
1 oz. birch leaves (*Betula alba*)
1 oz. yarrow (*Achillea millefolium*)
1 oz. juniper berries, crushed (*Juniperus communis*)
1 oz. wormwood (*Artemisia absinthium*)

Use: 1 tsp. per 1 cup boiling hot water. Steep 5 minutes and drink 1–3 cups per day before meals.

Formula 3

Restores and improves liver function.

1 oz. milk thistle (*Sylibum marianum*)
1 oz. dandelion root (*Taraxacum off.*)
1 oz. horehound (*Marrubium vulgare*)

Use: 1 tsp. per 1 cup boiling-hot water and steep for 15 minutes. Drink 3 cups per day before meals.

OLD-TIME WATER TREATMENTS THAT STIMULATE LIVER FUNCTION

European health spas such as Kitzbühl, Bad Neydharting, and Bad Tatzmannsdorf prescribe mud baths for liver and gallbladder ailments, while Bad Aussee and Bad Ischl (one of my favorites) are famous for their sulfur-rich, healing mineral water. Kneipp and other spas recommend herbal poultices and footbaths for patients suffering from liver ailments.

Don't despair if you can't visit any of those wonderful spas where healing is done the old-fashioned way. Instead, enjoy old-time water treatments in the privacy of your own home. A warm footbath and a warm compress placed over the abdomen is known to relieve discomfort and stimulate liver and gallbladder function. Both therapies, although simple, continue to enjoy popularity among holistically-oriented European doctors.

MONEY-SAVING HOME REMEDIES FOR LIVER AND GALLBLADDER AILMENTS

If you enjoy red beets and black radishes, indulge. These simple vegetables rejuvenate your liver.

Red beets are rich in vitamins and minerals, especially natural iron, and help detoxify and strengthen your liver. I often recommend a three-day beet fast (mono fast) to women with a sluggish metabolism. Instead of depleting your system, this fast provides plenty of vital nutrients that fortify your blood, stimulate digestion, promote regeneration of liver cells, and make you feel like a million.

Eat beets any way you like them—raw, boiled, pickled, or juiced—and for just a few cents per day, you can rejuvenate your liver. And please don't throw away the nutritious cooking water. If you don't like its taste (I love it), mix it with other juices. Your body will reward you for this tender, loving care by no longer causing the "monthly blues."

Black radish juice has aided liver and gallbladder ailments since ancient times. The Egyptians were fond of it, and famous men like the Greek historian Herodotus and the Roman Pliny the Younger praised its medicinal value. European herbals dating back to the Middle Ages recommend black radish as do holistically-oriented modern German medical doctors like Dr. Ludwig Wegener. Black radish, European medical history indicates, benefits a sluggish liver and gallbladder.

The gallbladder, a pear-shaped sack hanging between the lobes of the liver, is a reservoir of bile which is a liver secretion that serves both a digestive and excretory function. An inadequately functioning liver that cannot produce sufficient bile inevitably is the cause of digestive disorders.

Fresh black radish juice, Dr. Wegener says, improves liver and gallbladder function, stimulates gallbladder secretion, and prevents and heals inflammation.

Chemically speaking, raphanol, the main component of black radish, is a sulfur-containing oil that prevents and stops putrefactive bacteria. Black radish is also rich in potassium, calcium, iron, magnesium, phosphorus, and certainly sulfur, and is considered a mild antispasmodic, diuretic, and laxative. One to two tablespoons of juice taken before each meal quickly improve digestion.

A four-week juice cure benefits both the liver and gallbladder. Start by taking three to four ounces of black radish juice before breakfast for three days. Gradually increase amount to 12 to 16 ounces per day by drinking three to four ounces before each meal for one to two weeks. Gradually reduce the quantity and stop after three to four weeks, depending on results.

SIMPLE HERBAL TREATMENTS FOR DYSPEPSIA AND GALLBLADDER PROBLEMS

Dandelions deserve more than weedkillers. They are the most useful and easily available healing herb, and are indispensable to European natural health care. Fresh dandelion juice, prepared from chemical-free young leaves and roots, has long been recognized as a beneficial tonic for the entire digestive system, a tonic that stimulates liver action and improves gallbladder function.

Dr. M. Furlenmaier of Switzerland and other holistic health care practitioners recommend dandelion juice to activate the flow of bile and to prevent the formation of gallbladder stones. Taraxacerin, choline, niacin, vitamins A and C, levuline, inulin and pectin are dandelion's main ingredients and they are credited with stimulating the entire metabolism, detoxifying and strengthening the liver and kidneys. Dandelion root is also recognized for supporting pancreatic function.

Dandelion is one of the best natural diuretics. It is a mild laxative and tonic combining medicinal properties that are beneficial for the treatment of dyspepsia. European doctors recommend dandelion products as blood cleansers and to detoxify the digestive system.

In spring, young, unsprayed dandelion leaves make a healthy and delicious salad that was used generously by German folks during lean war and postwar years. Today, expensive greenhouse products or imported produce have replaced these wonderful healing greens, and instead of making the best of this weed, it is treated like a villain.

Dandelion roots and leaves make a healthy juice that is most effective for liver and gallbladder ailments. Drink 2–3 tablespoons of juice daily.

Extract: Use 2 tablespoons of fresh chopped leaves and roots per 2 glasses of cold water. Soak overnight, strain, and drink throughout the day.

Tea: Add 1–2 teaspoons of chopped leaves and roots to 1 cup of water. Bring to a boil, remove from heat, and soak for another 20 minutes. Strain and drink 1 cup in the mornings for 4–8 weeks. European health care professionals recommend that such a blood cleansing tonic be taken each spring when dandelions abound.

AN ANCIENT REMEDY THAT STIMULATES THE FLOW OF BILE (OR HOW TO LIVE WITHOUT A GALLBLADDER)

The herb, peppermint (*Mentha piperita*), enjoyed popularity among Oriental healers for thousands of years and was brought to Europe by missionaries. All mint species are useful medicinally but *Mentha piperita*, also called English Mint, is richest in essential oils. The American-grown species is the most valuable of all peppermint plants with good amounts of oils that yield up to 50% menthol, which is known for its antispasmodic, calming, and antiseptic properties. Menthol, peppermint's active ingredient, is eliminated via liver and gallbladder; it activates their function and stimulates the secretion of bile ninefold.

If you have had gallbladder surgery, you will benefit from peppermint tea. We generally recommend one cup of peppermint tea with each meal, plus necessary enzymes and bile (two tablets with each meal), and a daily intake of one teaspoon of lecithin, 25,000 International Units (I.U.) of vitamin A, 400 I.U. of vitamin E, 400 I.U. of vitamin D, plus generous amounts of acidophilus milk or yogurt. For cooking, use safflower oil rather than solid fats because vegetable oils are more readily absorbed. Eat small meals frequently and the first improvement you will notice is a softer stool, indicating that sufficient bile has been obtained.

PREVENTING GALLBLADDER COLIC, THE OLD-FASHIONED WAY

For centuries, European folk healers favored wormwood (*Artemisia absinthium*). Its products have long been recommended in the treatment of digestive disorders, particularly gallbladder colic, but just recently German health care professionals acknowledged the therapeutic value of this medicinal herb. Wormwood tea or tincture is now used to prevent and treat gallbladder colic. One cup of wormwood tea or 20 drops of tincture taken in hot water "relaxes" gallbladder activity and prevents painful colic.

Use ½ teaspoon herb per 1 cup hot water. Steep 10 minutes, strain and drink 1 cup to prevent gallbladder colic. (*Note:* Wormwood should be taken in small doses over a short period only.)

To prevent gallbladder colic, a hot oat straw compress placed over the liver and gallbladder area is recommended in addition to drinking tea or diluted tincture.

Use: Boil 1 cup of coarsely chopped oat straw in water, strain, and place oat straw into linen cloth. Apply warm. Use liquid to reheat compress.

AN UPDATED CUSTOMARY DIET PLAN
THAT REDUCES CHOLESTEROL

If your cholesterol level is low (200 or less), your chances of living to a healthy, ripe, old age are very good. Dutch medical doctors recently examined the blood of one hundred 90-year-olds, who were fairly active individuals, relatively free of diseases generally associated with old age. The survey revealed that all of the people tested preferred eating small, wholesome meals. Ninety-eight percent were nonsmokers, and each one showed low cholesterol levels.

It has been proven over and over again that the amount of cholesterol circulating in the blood is associated with heart diseases. Cholesterol levels above 300 milligram percent (mg %) increase your chances of suffering a heart attack and the higher the level, the greater the odds. Each year, one million Americans die from heart attacks, and at least half (or about 1,200 persons a day) die suddenly, within 24 hours of the first symptom of cardiac arrest. Many of these unfortunate deaths can be avoided.

Eliminating foods such as butter, eggs, lard, whole milk, cheese, cream, shellfish, and certain kinds of meat reduces cholesterol intake, yet this does not necessarily lower cholesterol levels substantially. Treatment is somewhat more complicated.

The liver synthesizes cholesterol in impressive amounts, and blood-fat levels need to be attacked from all directions. A fiber-rich diet is a must, as it forces the liver to convert cholesterol into bile salts, which are then excreted via the feces.

Lecithin plays an essential role in the reduction of blood fats. European doctors have long been aware of its relationship to elevated blood fats. Lecithin, a much-needed emulsifying agent normally produced by the liver to control cholesterol and other fats, aids patients suffering from atherosclerosis, a condition characterized by high blood cholesterol and low levels of lecithin. Lecithin supplementation has been especially beneficial to patients who have suffered heart attacks and strokes, or have cerebral atherosclerosis. The use of cold-pressed safflower and sunflower oils will also help to bring down cholesterol levels by aiding the body in its natural lecithin production.

Other nutrients involved in cholesterol regulation are B-12, biotin, choline, pangamic acid, and possibly inositol, all of which must be present to prevent accumulation of fat in the liver. Magnesium is also essential to keep blood cholesterol levels down and to prevent heart attacks.

Artichokes (*Cynara scolymus*) are more than a gourmet vegetable. Medicinally, the leaves and roots of artichokes are used to improve liver, gallbladder, and kidney function and aid the reduction of blood fats such as cholesterol and triglycerides. In France, Italy, Germany, and other European countries, artichoke juice or extract is a popular natural remedy that has proven useful in the treatment of atherosclerosis and the lowering of blood fats.

After my father's death, my mother suddenly developed frightening cholesterol and triglyceride levels. Medication didn't work—besides, mother had always been against taking drugs anyhow. We developed a high-roughage, largely vegetarian diet for her that included 2–3 tablespoons of bran plus plenty of wheat germ. This was supplemented with a high-potency vitamin B-complex, extra B-6 and B-12, multivitamin and multimineral supplements, 2,000 mg of chelated magnesium, 1,000 mg of vitamin C, and 400 I.U. of vitamin E. She took six tablespoons of lecithin daily, drank one cup of artichoke juice twice daily, and started a moderate exercise program. Today, her cholesterol and triglyceride levels are fairly normal (and have been for some time now) and by the time you read this, Mother will be a healthy 72 years old and still going strong. (Thank you, Mother!)

TRADITIONAL HERBAL REMEDIES
THAT STRENGTHEN YOUR HEART

Hawthorn (*Crataegus oxyacantha*) is a remarkable and most effective herbal cardiac tonic. It normalizes blood pressure (whether high or low) by regulating heart action and strengthening a weak heart muscle. In

Germany, old-fashioned hawthorn preparations are used to treat myocarditis (inflammation of the heart muscle), angina pectoris, atherosclerosis, nervous heart problems (irregular heartbeat and pulse, difficulty of breathing), and other nervous conditions. It is often prescribed as a preventive remedy for old people and given to individuals with a history of heart disease. European doctors also employ it to prevent cardiac arrest and to avoid digitalis therapy. Hawthorn preparations can be taken over months or years without causing unwanted side effects.

To make hawthorn tea, use 1–2 teaspoons of hawthorn flowers and/or leaves, add to 1 cup boiling-hot water (do not boil), and steep for 10 minutes. Drink 2–3 cups daily, hot or cold.

An old and popular German cardiac preparation is hawthorn and bean juice. (If you have a garden and a juicer, make your own cardiac tonic.) Hawthorn juice strengthens the heart muscle while bean juice acts as a diuretic that mildly stimulates the kidneys and aids the entire metabolism. Together, these traditional herbal remedies revive an overworked heart.

Use: Take 1 tablespoon 3–4 times daily with ½ cup of water about 15 minutes before meals. Children and old, sickly people should take 1 teaspoon 3–4 times per day.

Herbal Cardiac Formula for Nervous Heart Ailments

1 oz. hawthorn flowers (*Crataegus oxyacantha*)
1 oz. " leaves (")
1 oz. lemon balm (*Melissa off.*)
1 oz. oat straw (*Avena sativa*)

Use 1–2 teaspoons per 1 cup boiling-hot water, steep 10 minutes, and drink 2 cups during the day or before bedtime.

Old-Fashioned Herbal Formula for Angina Pectoris

1 oz. arnica flowers (*Arnica montana*)
1 oz. valerian root (*Valeriana off.*)
1 oz. malva leaves (*Malva sylvestris*). Use fresh leaves if possible.
1 oz. lemon balm (*Melissa off.*)
1 oz. rosmarin (*Rosmarinus off.*)
1 oz. hawthorn berries (*Crataegus oxyacantha*)

Use 2 teaspoons of herbal mixture per ½ cup of cold water. Soak overnight, bring to quick boil, and steep for 5 minutes. Drink ½ to 1 cup in small doses throughout the day.

Or, you may try rosmarin wine, an old-time favorite heart tonic that is effective, delicious, and simple to make.

Soak 3 oz. of rosmarin leaves in 1 quart white wine for four days. Filter and drink ¼ to ½ glass per day.

NATURAL TREATMENTS FOR KIDNEY AILMENTS

Do yourself a favor and be good to your kidneys. Your well-being depends on them.

Each day, five to seven liters of blood are cleansed about 300 times by your kidneys, and by the time you are 70, around 35 million liters of blood will have been detoxified by these relatively small, bean-shaped organs. Healthy kidneys throw off waste, prevent the body from dehydration, and keep it from becoming too acid or alkaline. Inadequately functioning kidneys allow toxic substances to pass into the blood, causing a life-threatening condition called toxemia. Kidney failure quickly causes death through poisoning.

A recent report published in the European medical journal, *Selecta*, indicates that inflammation of the kidneys is mainly the result of pain-killer abuse. According to a Swiss study, the danger of analgesics (painkillers) cannot be ignored or denied. Over ten years, a group of women who frequently used painkilling drugs were studied and compared to female non-drug users. Twelve percent of the drug users died of kidney failure. Their overall death rate was three times higher than that of the non-drug using women.

Kidney diseases are often accompanied by acute nutritional deficiencies similar to those found in patients with atherosclerosis. Restoring vital nutrients is an essential part of an otherwise simple, yet strict, treatment plan which follows:

• Cut out coffee, alcohol, and soft drinks. Sugar must be avoided. (British researchers indicate that sugar may contribute to stone formation.)

• Eat a wholesome diet, free of all artificial colorings, flavorings, preservatives, salt, and spices. Supplement it with vitamin A, B-complex, and magnesium. Use cold-pressed vegetable oil for cooking and supply most of your protein needs by eating yogurt, buttermilk, cottage cheese, eggs, and soy products, provided you can tolerate these foods.

• In severe cases, bedrest is necessary.

• The kidney area should be kept warm, and all medications should be eliminated if possible, but get your doctor's approval before you discontinue prescription drugs.

• Drink plenty of liquids to flush out the kidneys. For urine retention, drink uva ursi tea (see section on "Natural Diuretics" later in this chapter). Rosehip (*Rosa canina L.*) or peppermint tea (*Mentha piperita*) are mild diuretics which are useful for individuals with mildly elevated blood pressures.

The following century-old European herbal formulas have been useful in the treatment of kidney inflammation (pyelitis) and Bright's disease, including nephritis.

Herbal Formula That Aids Inflammation of the Kidneys

1 oz. birch leaves (*Betula alba*)
1 oz. speedwell (*Veronica officinalis*)
1 oz. European goldenrod (*Solidago Virgo-aurea*)
1 oz. rosehips (*Rosa canina*)
1 oz. parsley seeds (*Petroselinum sativum*)
1 oz. rosmarin (*Rosmarinus officinalis*)

Use 4 tablespoons per 2 pints cold water, soak for 2–3 hours, bring to quick boil, remove from heat, and steep for 5–10 minutes. Strain and drink unsweetened throughout the day.

Old-Fashioned Herbal Tea for Kidney Ailments

2 oz. European goldenrod (*Solidago Virgo-aurea*)
1 oz. restharrow (*Ononis spinosa*)
1 oz. birch leaves (*Betula alba*)
1 oz. elder flowers (*Sambuccus nigra*)
½ oz. juniper berries (*Juniperus communis*)

Add 2 teaspoons of herbal mixture to 1 cup boiling-hot water. Remove from heat and steep for 10 minutes. Strain and drink 1 cup each morning and noon.

HERBAL JUICES THAT STRENGTHEN BLADDER AND KIDNEY

Juice made from birch leaves (*Betula alba*) and shave grass (*Equisetum arvense*) strengthens kidneys and bladder, improves resistance, decreases inflammation, and is a mild and gentle diuretic that does not irritate the kidneys. If you suffer from recurring bladder and kidney ailments, do yourself a favor and get a juicer. Use fresh birch leaves and shave grass to make your own old-fashioned healing herbal juices. Take one tablespoon 3–4 times daily before meals. Children and sensitive individuals take 1 teaspoon 3–4 times daily with water (about ½ cup).

How Paul V. Flushed Away His Kidney Stones

Paul V. was a longtime patient of ours who frequently came to us seeking help for muscle tension and headaches. This time, the cause of it all was obvious. Paul was scheduled for surgery to remove troublesome kidney stones. He never had been hospitalized before, and he was frightened. The stones were small, medical tests indicated, but no treatment had been successful in eliminating them. Since the stones had triggered too many painful colic attacks, surgery seemed to be Paul's only hope.

Surgery was scheduled, but in the meantime we suggested a traditional German treatment that continues to be used prior to surgery when stones are small enough to be possibly and hopefully eliminated via the ureter.

Pimpernell (*Pimpinella saxifraga*) and rosehips (*Rosa canina*) stimulate the kidneys and promote elimination of gravel and stones, while birch leaves and restharrow are good diuretics that promote the flow of urine. Together, these old-fashioned herbal remedies can eliminate small stones and gravel.

Use: Soak overnight 2 tsp. of dried pimpernell rootstock and 2 tsp. of restharrow in 4 cups cold water. Strain and drink 1–2 tablespoons every hours.

Rosehip tea: Add 1 tsp. cut and sifted rosehips to 1 cup boiling-hot water. Remove from heat immediately and steep for 20 minutes. Drink liberal amounts throughout the day, preferably 2 cups or more every hour.

In addition, drink plenty of birch leaf tea. Use 2 handfuls of fresh or dried leaves per 2 cups boiling-hot water. Boil for 3–5 minutes and soak for 1½ hours. Strain and drink at least 1 cup each morning, noon and evening.

That may seem like a lot of fluid, but don't take shortcuts. Pour down all liquids, take 100 mg vitamin B-6 per day, and keep active. Exercise or walk, but stay near restrooms—you will need them. And watch out for your stones. If all goes well, you will quickly eliminate them.

Paul got lucky the third day, just before he was to report to the hospital. Talk about relief.

AVOIDING KIDNEY STONES

Paul saved some of the troublemakers (kidney stones) for analysis. You should try to do the same.

While foods are not the sole cause of stone formation, it is important to know what type of stones you are most likely to develop. If they are calciumoxalates, by all means avoid rhubarb, spinach, and figs. These oxalate-rich foods do contribute to the formation of such stones. Take magnesium; it prevents calcium formations. If you eat a calcium-rich diet or take calcium supplements, remember that this mineral needs to be balanced with magnesium. The proper calcium-magnesium ratio is 2:1, and if you are susceptible to stone formation, any imbalanced calcium is likely to be deposited in the form of stones. Therefore, increase your magnesium intake and, instead of causing trouble, calcium will benefit your health.

Stones formed of calcium combined with oxalic acid or phosphorus develop most rapidly when the urine is more alkaline. Stay away from all citrus fruits and their juices and eat more protein foods to create a more acidic urine. Stay away from all sugars and drink cranberry or grape juice. Take extra vitamin B-6 which helps to excrete oxalic acid.

Stones formed from urates are found in individuals who prefer a high-protein diet. To avoid stones, eliminate meat intake and drink restharrow tea regularly to stimulate uric acid excretion. Again, supplement your diet with magnesium to balance calcium levels, and eat and drink large amounts of fruits and vegetables and their juices. Citrus fruits are especially useful since they create an alkaline urine which keeps uric acid crystals in solution. If you are susceptible to sodium-urate stones, follow the gout diet given in Chapter 3.

Foods that benefit kidney ailments and help prevent stone formation are cucumbers, celery, and parsley—mild diuretics that were used in ancient Greece to strengthen kidneys and bladder.

Exercise. Perspiration promotes elimination of waste products from the body—and less waste means less work for the kidneys.

TRADITIONAL REMEDIES FOR URINARY INFECTIONS

A few years back, our daughter suddenly developed a bladder infection that caused her quite a bit of discomfort. Instead of subjecting her to antibiotic treatment, we successfully used old-time, natural remedies. Within three days, she was symptom-free as was indicated by urine tests and her general well-being. We have since recommended this treatment to patients with good results.

1. Take 2–3 garlic capsules 3–4 times daily. Garlic is a natural antibiotic that fights invading bacteria without upsetting a healthy intestinal flora.
2. Drink 2–3 cups of a natural herbal diuretic tea per day (see "Natural Diuretics" section, to follow in this chapter).
3. Drink plenty of cranberry and/or grape juice to promote urine acidity that helps retard bacterial growth.
4. Avoid all citrus fruits and their juices as they cause urine alkalinity, which promotes bacterial growth. The smell of ammonia in urine indicates severe alkalinity. Reduce carbohydrate intake and eliminate all sugar.
5. Take 20,000 I.U. of vitamin A (adults take 50,000 I.U.), 200–400 I.U. of vitamin E (adults take 400–800 I.U.), 2–3 high-potency B-complex supplements, and 2,000 mg of vitamin C (adults more) until symptoms disappear.
6. Keep bladder and kidney area warm. Hot packs ease discomfort.
7. Rest.

We improved this natural therapy for Betty K., who was hospitalized with a severe bladder infection that had prevented her from urinating for several days. A catheter had been inserted once and the procedure was scheduled again. Since medical treatments had obviously brought little relief, Betty K.'s husband, a former patient of ours, came seeking advice. We told him about the above treatment for urinary infections and recommended uva ursi leaves (*Arctostaphylos uva-ursi*) as a diuretic. This medicinal herb (see section on "Natural Diuretics") is very effective in the relief of bladder and kidney infections. European doctors have successfully employed it since the eighteenth century and folk healers recommended it long before that time.

Betty K. drank two cups of this bitter-tasting brew throughout the next day, and don't ask how her husband got the doctor to approve this and all the other supplements. It wasn't easy, but it was worth every effort. During the following night Betty K. was able to urinate, and when the surprised urologist came to see her, he even encouraged Betty to continue this natural program. Thanks to an open-minded physician who did not simply discard traditional remedies, Betty K. quickly regained her health.

NATURAL DIURETICS

European health care providers consider uva ursi to be (*Arctostaphylos uva-ursi*) *the* most effective herbal diuretic. It promotes urination and has a definite healing effect on kidneys and bladder. This widely recognized medicinal herb is not a diuretic in the pharmaceutical sense, however. It actually strengthens the urinary tract, and if given in small doses (one tablespoon three times daily taken over six weeks) uva ursi is known to correct bed-wetting.

With this medicinal herb, more is *not* better. On the contrary, overdoses may cause vomiting. To aid urinary infection, soak 1–2 tablespoons of dried leaves in 2 cups cold water. Bring to a quick boil, strain, and drink 1–2 cups per day until symptoms disappear. (*Note:* The herb's main component, arbutin, causes brown discoloration of the urine, which is nothing to be concerned about.)

Birch leaves (*Betula alba, B. pubescens* and others), which have been mentioned in ancient Sanskrit writings, have been recognized for their medicinal value ever since man learned to treat his ailments through natural remedies. The Barbarians, Greeks, and Romans were all fond of this healing herb, as were the Chinese, who have employed it since the tenth century. Modern European phytotherapists continue to endorse this useful herb, which particularly enjoys popularity among the Scandinavians, who employ it for arthritic aches and pains (see Chapter 3).

Clearly a powerful diuretic that also stimulates perspiration, birch leaf remedies do not irritate kidneys and bladder. European natural health care providers chiefly prescribe its use in the treatment of kidney ailments and related skin problems, arthritic ailments, gout, and edemas.

Steep 4 teaspoons fresh or dried birch leaves in 2 cups hot water for 10 minutes, strain, and drink up to 2 cups per day.

Foods such as asparagus, celery root, fennel root, and parsley make mild diuretics. Cut and dried, they may be used as natural diuretic teas during winter. Rosehip is another mild diuretic that adds wonderful flavor to any tea.

To make tea from dried vegetables, roots, or herbs, mix together 1 oz. of each dried plant and steep 1 teaspoon of this mixture in ½ to 1 cup boiling-hot water for 5 to 10 minutes. Strain and drink 1 cup per day.

Natural Herbal Diuretic Tea Formula That Strengthens Bladder and Kidneys

   1 oz. birch leaves (*Betula alba*)
   1 oz. dandelion root (*Taraxacum off.*)
   1 oz. rosehips (*Rosa canina*)
   1 oz. licorice root (*Glycyrrhiza glabra*)
   ½ oz. uva ursi (*Arctostaphylos uva-ursi*)
   Use 1 teaspoon per 1 cup boiling-hot water. Steep 5–10 minutes, strain, and drink 1–2 cups per day.

****

References:

Cheraskin, E., M.D., D.M.D.; Clark, J.W., D.D.S.; Ringsdorf, W.M., Jr., D.M.D. *Diet and Disease.* Keats Publ., 1968.

Cheraskin, E., M.D., D.M.D.; Ringsdorf, W.M., Jr., D.M.D. *Predictive Medicine.* Keats Publ., 1973.

Fredericks, Carlton, Ph.D. *New and Complete Nutrition Handbook.* Major Books, 1976.

Freise, Eduard, Dr. *Der Drogist.* Von Morgenstern, F., Dr., Band 1 & 2, Killinger Verlag, (no date).

Furlenmaier, M., M.D. *Wunderwelt der Heilpflanzen.* Zurich: Rheingauer Verlag, Schwitter Holding AG, 1978.

Goerz, Heinz. *Gesundheit durch Heilkraeuter.* W. Moeller Verlag, 1974.

Heinerman, John. *Science of Herbal Medicine*. By-World, 1979.

Kugler, Hans J., Ph.D. *Dr. Kugler's Seven Keys to a Longer Life*. New York: Stein and Day, 1978.

Kunz-Bircher, Ruth. *The Bircher-Benner Health Guide*. Woodbridge Press, 1980.

Lindt, Inge. *Naturheilkunde, Heilkraeuter und ihre Anwendung, Krankheiten und ihre Behandlung*. Buch und Zeit, 1977.

Lust, John B., N.D. *The Herb Book*. Lust Publ., 1974.

Pfeiffer, Carl C. M.D., Ph.D. *Mental and Elemental Nutrients*. Keats Publ., 1975.

Reuben, David, M.D. *The Save Your Life Diet*. New York: Random House, 1975.

Schauenberg, P.; Paris, F. *BLV Bestimmungsbuch Heilpflanzen*. BLV, 1978.

Spoerke, David G. Jr. *Herbal Medications*. Woodbridge Press Publ., 1980.

Stage, Wolfgang, M.D. *Das Kneipp Taschenbuch*. Ullstein, 1968.

Steen, Edwin B., Ph.D.; Montagu, Ashley, Ph.D. *Anatomy and Physiology*. Barnes & Noble, 1959.

Williams, Roger, Jr., Ph.D. *Nutrition Against Disease*. Int. Institute of Natural Sciences, CA.

Apotheken Umschau, Vol. 1A, 1980.

Der Wegweiser, Vol. 6, 1979.

————— .   Vol. 4, 1980.

————— .   Vol. 8, 1980.

————— .   Vol. 15, 1980.

————— .   Vol. 16, 1980.

Reform Rundschau, Vol. 8, 1979.

————— .   Vol. 9, 1979.

————— .   Vol. 10, 1979.

————— .   Vol. 1, 1980.

————— .   Vol. 2, 1980.

————— .   Vol. 3, 1980.

————— .   Vol. 4, 1980.

————— .   Vol. 6, 1980.

The ACA Journal of Chiropractic. April 1976, pp. 46-48.

5

Old-Time Treatments Prevent and Relieve Glandular Problems

UNDERSTANDING BODY SIGNALS

You haven't felt well for a long time. Worse yet, you don't even remember what feeling in tiptop condition is like, and the numerous medical check-ups you've had reveal nothing. According to your doctor you are in good health, yet despite this clean bill of health you still feel lousy.

The truth is, most doctors are concerned only about the classical signs of disease, and as long as your symptoms don't fit textbook patterns you are considered healthy, or even worse, you are labeled a hypochondriac or psychopath, especially if you happen to be a woman.

Well, don't wait until you are recognized as a classical medical case. Listen to your body signals, and if there is any indication that your well-being is less than perfect, pay attention and do what our forefathers did—aid the body in healing itself. It can be done.

To be easily tired and depressed is not normal. Health is feeling good, and anything less than that should be acknowledged as your body's way of telling you that something is out of tune. Feeling less than perfect means your body needs extra attention, and any adverse body symptom is a cry for help.

This help, your doctor insists, should come from a psychiatrist or psychologist because all your symptoms are purely mental. So you went to an analyst. You faced your hidden problems, and you now understand yourself better than ever. But you are still plagued with depression, nervousness, and other symptoms. In short, little has changed.

Since nobody seems to understand your problems, perhaps it is time to take matters into your own hands. Learn more about yourself. Get a diary. Each day write down how you felt, what you ate, and what your day was like. After a few weeks or months, see if you notice some kind of a pattern or relationship developing. You may find that you are more susceptible to depression before your period, if you are a woman, that stress causes you to react, or that certain foods contribute to your problems. You may notice that on one day, problems hardly bother you at all, while on other days, every little problem causes anxiety or depression.

If that sounds familiar, take a good look at your glandular system. It may need a little more attention.

Traditional and modern nutritional therapies can successfully correct glandular imbalances. After all, until recently, synthetic hormones were unknown and diseases of the endocrine system had to be treated naturally. Old-fashioned remedies may not bring instant results, but they can regulate hormonal imbalances and assure you a happy, healthy life.

MORE ABOUT HORMONES

Hormones are organic chemical compounds produced by glands of the endocrine system to help regulate and correlate body activities. Glands which comprise the endocrine system are: the pituitary, the thyroid, the parathyroid, the adrenals, the pancreas, the testes, and the ovaries.

The hormones produced by the testes, ovaries, and the adrenal cortex are steroids, which are thought to be derived from cholesterol, while all the other hormones are nitrogen compounds derived from proteins.

Since nerve impulses and chemical reactions all influence glandular secretion, specific foods and herbs, which supply nutrients and similar chemical substances, *can* influence hormonal activity.

Hormones are potent substances, and an over- or undersupply of them greatly affects the body as a whole. Hormones control growth, development, maturation, reproduction, energy metabolism, and more, and to a great degree, influence emotional well-being.

If your doctor gives you a clean bill of health and you still feel less than adequate, and if, despite having an understanding partner, your sex life is less than fulfilling and your emotional state leaves much to be desired, take a good look at your glandular system and take some action today.

A SIMPLE TEST HELPS REVEAL
THYROID DISORDERS

You feel run-down and depressed. You suffer from recurring headaches, are the first to catch colds and flus, your skin is a constant source of problems, and hair loss seems abnormal. Or, perhaps you can't wind down from your hectic pace, have difficulty sleeping, and are extremely irritable? Take a good look at your thyroid. It may be the troublemaker.

Since the thyroid is instrumental in regulating energy, an increase or decrease in hormonal secretion directly reflects on the basal metabolic rate. In the *hyper*thyroid patient, the basal temperature is higher than normal, while the *hypo*thyroid patient typically runs low temperatures. Thus, the basal temperature can serve as a simple guide to determine thyroid function. Normal values for underarm temperature are in the range of 97.8 to 98.2 degrees Fahrenheit. Temperatures below 97.8 may indicate a low thyroid function, while a basal temperature above 98.2 may indicate hyperfunction.

Unfortunately, diagnostic accuracy is rarely 100%, and while the basal temperature test was found to be nearly 80% correct (which makes it as good a diagnostic test as any), low readings can be influenced by other hormonal dysfunctions such as a pituitary or an adrenal deficiency. In the presence of infections, temperature readings can certainly lead to misinterpretation.

The basal temperature test as recommended by Broda O. Barnes, M.D., is simple. Women past the menopause and men can take it any given morning, but menstruating women need to consider their menstrual cycle, which causes fluctuations in temperature. Therefore, it is best for women to start taking the basal temperature test a few days after the onset of menstruation and continue to take it for a week to ten days.

To receive accurate readings, you should take your temperature in the morning immediately after you wake up. Don't go to the bathroom before you take the test because the slightest physical activity will raise your temperature, leading to false results. As a matter of fact, you shouldn't even shake down the thermometer. Do that the night before and place it within your reach.

OLD AND NEW TREATMENTS FOR
HYPOTHYROIDISM

Your temperature is consistently low but your doctor, who ran a thyroid checkup, insists there is nothing wrong. According to the blood test your thyroid functions just fine.

Don't panic. You are not a hypochondriac ready for the funny farm. Considering all circumstances, the test we just discussed is not misleading you and neither is your blood test.

The problem lies somewhere else. Medical diagnosis and evaluation of all tests, including blood chemistry profiles, are concerned strictly with acute disease. Anything else is considered nonexistent. You may have all the classical symptoms of hypothyroidism—lowered body temperature; slowed heart rate; muscle weakness; sensitivity to colds and infections; dry skin; dry, thin hair; brittle fingernails; and slow wound healing. You may also complain about fatigue, apathy, and chronic constipation, but if your blood test does not reveal obvious thyroid dysfunction, you are considered healthy.

Take a look at the situation's bright side: if mild cases would be medically acknowledged, drug treatment and surgery would reach more epidemic proportions, leading to increased drug abuse and more unnecessary surgery.

You know your health problems better than anyone. Start paying closer attention to your body signals—and start helping yourself.

All hypothyroid patients respond quickly to nutritional therapy, and while it has been commonly accepted that hypothyroidism is a lifelong condition, European studies indicate that this does not have to be the case. Hypothyroidism can be corrected.

Consider the case of Emma R., who hadn't felt good in years. According to her, she was basically "getting by." When she came to our clinic, she simply wanted us to take care of her recurrent headaches and recommend a sensible diet that "wouldn't mess me up even more."

Like many borderline hypothyroid patients, Emma had accepted feeling inadequate. "I am not complaining about being tired all the time," she said. "I guess that's the way it is with me." She often made fun of herself. "I was born tired," she once said, "and don't make an appointment for me next week, unless you want to treat a bad witch. My period, you know." Emma joked about her increasing disinterest in sex, but deep down she was scared. Not only did she feel her life slipping away; her marriage was at stake.

Emma knew her menstrual cycle affected her emotionally and physically, and she was able to predict when she would come down with a cold or the flu. She used to take vitamins, but since they didn't seem to help, she basically had given up on nutritional supplements.

Despite all her problems, Emma was a pleasant person with a good sense of humor. Yet, her life was overshadowed by depressions that hit her regularly "like a ton of bricks."

We asked her to take the basal temperature test, and along with it, record her mood swings and energy levels. The results were not surprising. Her body temperature fluctuated dramatically and frequently fell below normal. During the critical premenstrual times, when she was highly susceptible to depression and infection, Emma's basal temperature was below 97 degrees Fahrenheit.

Since hypothyroidism is often accompanied by anemia, glucose intolerance, and high cholesterol and triglyceride levels, we also evaluated Emma's blood chemistry. Her cholesterol level was close to 300 mg/100 ml., her glucose levels indicated a hypoglycemic condition, and her adrenal and liver functions were somewhat impaired. Anemia was not a problem yet, though mild symptoms were obvious. The thyroid function test revealed borderline hypothyroidism. A hair analysis indicated low levels of copper, chromium, and magnesium and high levels of zinc, all of which are considered typical symptoms of hypothyroidism.

To stimulate the patient's metabolism, we temporarily put her on a carbohydrate-restricted diet that included only those fruits and vegetables that are considered low in carbohydrates, such as asparagus, cucumber, lettuce, tomatoes, beets, carrots, strawberries, blackberries, and grapefruit. The diet, which is patterned after Dr. Broda O. Barnes's hypothyroid program, contains about 50 grams of carbohydrate, 70 grams of protein, and some fat, totalling up to about 1,300 calories per day. On this diet, no patient needs to endure hunger pains or energy loss. On the contrary, patients generally feel better and experience a steady weight loss. Since the diet supplies practically no grains, it is supplemented with three teaspoons of bran to aid digestion and cholesterol breakdown, plus the following nutritional supplements:

- Multivitamin and mineral supplement, one tablet daily.
- 10,000 I.U. of vitamin A in addition to the 25,000 I.U. found in the multivitamin and mineral tablet, and 2,000 mg of vitamin C were given to improve resistance to infection.
- High-potency vitamin B-complex, three to five daily. Since all of the B-vitamins are readily lost, we advised her not to take them all at once, but to take one tablet with each meal or snack. Since many of the B-vitamins are involved in the metabolism of carbohydrates, fats, and proteins, such supplementation improves digestion and energy metabolism.
- Additional vitamin B-6 and 1,200 mg of lecithin were given to reduce cholesterol and triglyceride levels.
- Take 1 teaspoon hypoallergenic amino acid powder 20 minutes before each meal to support hormone and enzyme production.
- To further improve digestion, we recommended digestive enzymes containing pepsin and hydrochloric acid, along with manganese,

which activates enzyme activity and improves the utilization of vitamin C and the B vitamins.

• To avoid anemia, a daily intake of 50 mg of chelated iron and 50 micrograms of vitamin B-12 was recommended.

• To support liver function and red blood cell formation, red beets and red beet juice were part of Emma's diet.

• Since an iodine deficiency often is the cause of hypothyroidism, one teaspoon of kelp, which is more readily absorbed than potassium or sodium iodide, was part of the supplemental program.

• Because a vitamin E deficiency decreases iodine absorption, 400 I.U. of vitamin E were recommended, along with 50 mg of chelated chromium to improve glucose tolerance.

To support the thyroid glands and the adrenals, glandular supplements were included in the program, and since recent European medical studies indicate that fluoride and chloride intake possibly inhibit thyroid function, we told Emma to avoid all sources of these organochemical compounds, including tap water. Salicylates also depress hormonal output; therefore, Emma was advised to avoid all aspirin sources. Because all cabbages, including cauliflower and broccoli, are possible thyroid inhibitors, these vegetables were excluded from her diet. Rutabagas, turnips, soyflower, and raw peanuts were eliminated for the same reason.

It was difficult for Emma to follow this extensive nutritional program, but since she didn't have a better alternative she pledged to stick with this program, at least for two months.

Within a week, Emma reported a noticeable improvement in energy and emotional stability, even though it was time for her "regular low." After three months, Emma admitted to "feeling like new," and commented that her husband noticed her improved interest in life and sex. A follow-up blood test was taken which revealed considerable improvement in all areas, and though we did not emphasize weight loss during the initial treatment period, Emma experienced a steady weight loss of between one-half to one pound per week, which her husband called "an unexpected bonus."

Emma continues to be on a modified nutritional program. Her carbohydrate intake has been increased because losing weight is no longer a necessity and today, Emma is a happy and energetic woman who takes a new interest in her family and her community by volunteering for work on the local "Meals on Wheels" program.

OLD-FASHIONED REMEDIES FOR
HYPERTHYROIDISM

Hyperthyroidism, also called Grave's disease, refers to a state of heightened thyroid activity associated with an overproduction of thyroid hormone caused by insufficient enzyme production. Accumulating hormones cause a "speedy metabolism" with resulting weight loss, extreme nervousness, and an inability to rest and relax. The typical hyperthyroid patient appears to be restless or hyperactive, yet his energy level is often low. He may complain about sudden onsets of fatigue and weakness that may result in tremors. His pulse rate is fast, heart sounds are intensified, and the basal temperature is above normal, enabling the hyperthyroid patient to easily tolerate the cold. A shortened menstrual cycle, missed periods, or infertility are symptoms often associated with acute and borderline hyperthyroidism in women.

Consider the case of Grace U., who didn't think that stress was responsible for her nervous ailments. She rather insisted that her "nerves play tricks that cause problems."

Grace had many of the typical symptoms of a hyperthyroid patient. She complained about being jittery, jumpy, and irritable, and while she often felt extremely tired, a restful sleep seemed hard to come by. She suffered from frequent headaches, her menstruation was irregular, and though she and her husband had tried everything, "including fancy medical tests that showed we are normal," conceiving a child seemed impossible.

Since a blood test revealed borderline hyperthyroid function, we decided to modify a special nutritional program that has long been emphasized by German and other European health care practitioners, and Grace agreed to give it a try. Indeed, it has been established that simple dietary changes can quickly improve symptoms of hyperthyroidism and can prevent the need for surgical removal of toxic thyroid glands.

To reduce Grace's racy metabolism, we immediately placed her on a vegetarian diet, supplying eggs, milk products, and whole grains to satisfy protein needs, and plenty of fresh fruits and vegetables rich in nutrients, fiber, and natural enzymes. Raw peanuts, soyflower, turnips, rutabagas, and cabbages such as broccoli and cauliflowers, known to inhibit thyroid hormone production, were part of the diet. Ample amounts of grape juice and an herbal tea mixture containing milk thistle, peppermint, and dandelion root were recommended to aid liver and kidney function.

Since proper liver function helps regulate enzyme synthesis and hormonal activity, liver glandulars were part of this nutritional program. The following supplements were recommended to further regulate thyroid function and meet this patient's individual nutritional needs.

Dolomite, 6 tablets daily

High-potency B-complex, 1 with each meal

Digestive enzymes, 1–2 with each meal

A high-potency multi-vitamin/mineral supplement containing 25,000 I.U. of vitamin A, to be taken twice daily

Vitamin E, 800 I.U. daily

Vitamin C, 2 grams daily

Chiropractic adjustments have successfully relieved her headaches, and within two months, Grace noticed a tremendous improvement in her overall condition. A follow-up blood test showed that her thyroid function had returned to normal, and after approximately five months on the outlined nutritional program, Grace became pregnant. Again, we modified her diet to meet the demands of pregnancy, and now, as you read this, Grace and her husband are proud parents.

SIMPLE DIETARY CHANGES EFFECTIVELY COPE WITH ADDISON'S DISEASE

Since the adrenals, which rise from atop the kidneys, pour out numerous hormones (adrenalin, epinephrin, and cortisone), adrenal exhaustion, such as Addison's disease, seriously impairs the body's response to stress and injury. Adrenal insufficiency impairs muscular activity, the body's salt metabolism, reproductive activity, kidney function, the basal metabolism, carbohydrate metabolism, and affects the nervous system. Typical symptoms of adrenal exhaustion caused by inhibited hormone production are extreme fatigue, apathy, and muscle weakness.

It has been well established that adrenal problems cause an imbalance in the electrolytes. Generally, salt reduction is admirable unless adrenal insufficiency is suspected or has been medically dignosed. Then, salt consumption is necessary to restore proper mineral balance. A blood test reveals whether potassium is needed in addition to salt (sodium), but potassium supplementation should be used only temporarily with control exercised by a capable health care provider. A diet rich in raw fruits and vegetables further helps create this proper balance and supplies other needed nutrients and enzymes. Green, leafy vegetables, wheat germ, brewer's yeast and glandular supplements should be part of the nutritional program for supporting the adrenal system.

Stress increases the body's nutritional demands for the B-vitamins by many times. Pantothenic acid, vitamin B2, B6, and C requirements are especially high during adrenal insufficiency, and if supplied generously, production of adrenal hormones can resume normally within 24 hours. Vitamin C can prevent stress reactions and actually detoxify harmful substances formed during stress.

Animals who manufacture vitamin C within their own systems are better able to withstand stress, and experiments with guinea pigs exposed to severe colds revealed that a mild vitamin C deficiency causes adrenals to hemorrhage, resulting in death. Those animals receiving massive doses of vitamin C were able to withstand stress situations without problems.

While Addison's disease is a comparatively rare condition, mild degrees of adrenal insufficiency due to prolonged stress are relatively common. A typical hypoglycemic diet, supplying antistress factors as outlined above and an increased salt intake, is generally all that is needed to improve adrenal function and counterbalance the individual's reaction to stress.

WHY I EAT SIX MEALS A DAY

During my teenage years, hypoglycemia was never diagnosed. This disabling condition was not understood, and therefore did not exist by medical standards.

Hypoglycemia was prevalent, however, and I can testify to that. Due to Audrey Hepburn's smashing success, being thin was the goal of most teenagers of the late Fifties, and dieting was definitely "in." We all loathed being of average weight; we hated any trace of baby fat. We wanted to be skinny and bony, and adored what Mother called "the hungry look." Needless to say, we suffered to achieve it. Dieting, or should I say, fasting, didn't agree with me. Fasting caused weakness, gross irritability, immense headaches, and when stress piled up, I simply blacked out. Since these fainting spells often happened before important examinations, I quickly got a reputation for being an "actress," especially since doctors concluded I was "nervous but healthy." It is still embarrassing to think about, but after awhile, even I thought my health problems were caused by my wild imagination and fear of tests.

In a way, that was true, of course. Low blood sugar causes symptoms of stress such as tension, irritability, headache, and fatigue, and when stress levels increase, much potassium is lost in the urine and blackouts occur. Excess sodium causes water to be retained, which makes it difficult for the hypoglycemic patient to lose weight even while on a reducing diet. Modern research indicates that when potassium is part of the nutritional program of the hypoglycemic patient, blackouts and other unpleasant symptoms are prevented, and weight loss is more easily achieved.

It is well-known that all people suffering from glucose intolerance, including diabetes and hypoglycemia, benefit from eating frequent and small protein meals, and don't forget that meat is not the only source of protein. High-quality proteins are found in eggs, dairy products, and can be obtained by combining these with soy products, grains, nuts, and vegetable sources.

Hypoglycemia means low blood sugar, and although this may sound as if it indicates a need for dietary sugar, don't touch the stuff. Sugar is the hypoglycemic's worst enemy because refined carbohydrates (and sugar is pure carbohydrate) overstimulate the pancreas, causing excessive insulin secretion. Excessive insulin causes blood sugar to fall; it also changes most blood sugar into storage fat.

While it is difficult, if not impossible, for the hypoglycemic to fast, weight loss can be achieved. A high protein-low fat diet usually works best. Small meals should be eaten frequently, and the dieter is better off by limiting carbohydrates rather than calories. This way, hunger pains, fainting spells, irritability, etc., can be avoided.

To improve the hypoglycemic's condition it is important to support pancreatic function. This can be done by supplementing the diet with pancreatic enzymes, amino acids and ample amounts of the vitamin B-complex.

Bean pod tea or juice helps to regulate blood sugar levels, and this old-fashioned European remedy continues to be endorsed by German medical doctors with excellent results. Improving liver function (see Chapter 4) also reduces symptoms of hypoglycemia.

While a multiple vitamin-and-mineral supplement provides most needed nutrients, individual nutritional requirements need to be met. The Glucose Tolerance Factor (GTF), containing chromium, nicotinic acid, and three amino acids, is essential for insulin regulation and may be the underlying prerequisite for proper carbohydrate metabolism, without which hypoglycemia or diabetes develops.

It has been established that uncontrolled hypoglycemia can lead to diabetes; however, this does not indicate that hypoglycemia is a lifelong or life-threatening condition. On the contrary, it is easily controlled by dietary means, enabling the hypoglycemic patient to lead a normal, symptom-free life.

I can testify to that. After I had learned to meet my body's individual requirements, hypoglycemic symptoms gradually lessened, and while I generally eat six nutritious meals a day, I can now miss a meal or two—without experiencing any side effects. My blood sugar level is normal and I have no difficulty maintaining weight. I am healthy, though I remain on a hypoglycemic diet "because I am worth it."

SELF-HELP FOR DIABETICS

Dietary changes can alter the course of diabetes. This has been recognized since the nineteenth century, and modern research significantly added to this understanding.

More than 80% of adult diabetics are overweight at the time the disorder is diagnosed, and a great many have high levels of triglycerides—blood fats that correspond to sugar intake. Health problems that frequently complicate diabetes are atherosclerosis, cataracts, fatty liver, gangrene, overweight, and retinitis.

Basically, all diabetic individuals need to correct their weight problems and nutritional deficiencies. The use of simple sugars and alcohol has to be eliminated, and blood fat levels need to be further reduced by limiting all fat intake.

Most diabetics have high nutritional requirements for vitamins A, the B-complex, especially the B-vitamins B1, pantothenic acid, and biotin, and have unusually great needs for vitamin C.

Adelle Davis reports that an elderly attorney, who had taken 80 units of protamine-zinc insulin for ten years, increased his vitamin C intake to 4,000 milligrams (4 grams) per day to aid a prostate infection. As a result of his increased vitamin C intake, his physician had to reduce his insulin intake repeatedly and finally discontinue it.

Diabetics are frequently deficient in potassium and magnesium, and if atherosclerosis or gangrene is a threat, vitamin E and lecithin intake need to be increased. Chromium helps the body to better tolerate sugars, and pancreatic enzymes and amino acids support pancreatic function.

Medicinal herbs such as goat's-rue (*Galega officinalis*), fenugreek (*Trigonella foenum-graecum*), walnut leaves (*Juglans regia*), bilberry leaves (*Vaccinium myrtillus*), great burdock (*Arctium lappa*), bean pods (*Phaseolus vulgaris*), and great nettle leaves (*Urtica dioica*) help reduce blood sugar levels.

It is possible to reduce insulin dependency. German and other European pharmaceutical companies actually promote herbal formulas for the treatment of diabetes as much as they endorse insulin therapy.

My best friend, who had been on insulin therapy for two years, followed her doctor's suggestion to use a specific diabetic tea. This, plus a change in diet, slowly reduced her need for insulin and today she leads a normal, healthy life.

TRADITIONAL REMEDIES FOR CONTROLLING THE MONTHLY BLUES

Premenstrual tension and menstrual cramps can temporarily take the joy out of womanhood, and while female complaints are common, few women know how to eliminate these problems naturally. While drug treatment brings momentary relief, it does not remove underlying causes. As a result, menstruation problems return month after month.

When the thyroid is underactive, abnormal menstrual flow is often a problem because the thyroid hormones influence ovarian function. When thyroid function returns to normal, most likely menstruation returns to normal. Therefore, if your basal temperature indicates a thyroid condition, throw away your aspirins and improve your thyroid function instead.

Supporting liver function indirectly relieves female problems. The liver plays a role in the activation and inactivation of hormones, and is the actual storage place of iron and copper, minerals which are necessary for proper red blood cell formation.

The pituitary hormone (which stimulates ovarian function) and estrogen (the ovarian hormone) regulate the reproductive cycle. When amino acids, linoleic acid, the B vitamins, and vitamin E are deficient, these hormones cannot be synthesized. When estrogen is deficient, calcium absorption is inadquate, and menstrual cramps and nervous problems abound.

Therefore, Mother's old-time remedy makes sense. Before the start of your period drink plenty of milk (if you suffer from a milk allergy, use other calcium sources) and beet juice to obtain much-needed calcium, iron, potassium, and other nutrients. Eating beets will provide roughage and stimulate bowel movements.

When menstruation is difficult and painful, yarrow tea (*Achillea millefolium*) or juice helps eliminate spasms and increase the menstrual flow.

To make the tea, add 2–3 tablespoons of the herb to 1 pint hot water (do not boil). Steep for 15 minutes, strain, and drink 1 cup three times daily.

Yarrow juice can be made from the fresh herb, and according to the Swiss medical doctor Furlenmaier, 2–3 teaspoons of yarrow juice are to be taken daily with warm water or beef, chicken, or vegetable broth.

Yarrow sitz baths have been used for centuries by European folk healers to ease female problems and are still endorsed by German midwives to ease painful menstruation.

Lemon balm tea or extract may be considered Germany's herbal answer to Valium. Lemon balm (*Melissa officinalis*) remedies relax the nervous system, aid insomnia, and relieve all sorts of spasms, particularly those due to menstruation. Lemon balm extract (German: *Melissengeist*) is still found in every German drugstore and in most Germans' medicine cabinets.

Internally, lemon balm tea or extract relieves all spastic conditions, including tension headaches; externally, it soothes muscle pain.

Tea: add 2 teaspoons of leaves to 1 cup hot water and steep for 10 minutes. Strain and drink 1–3 cups per day. To induce sleep, drink 1 cup before bedtime in small doses, sweetened with honey.

Paracelsus and Lonicerus praised the medicinal value of lady's mantle (*Alchemilla vulgaris*), the herb many European women drink during the later part of pregnancy to ease childbirth. Sitz baths and douches are traditional European remedies for irregular periods, vaginal infections, and excessive vaginal discharge.

Tea: Use 1 teaspoon herb for 1 cup hot water. Steep 10 minutes, strain, and drink, 1–4 cups per day.

Sitz bath: Add 4 oz. of herb to 1 pint cold water. Bring to boil and simmer over low heat for 10 minutes. Strain and add to bath water, or use as wash.

To regulate menstruation, use the following herbal mixture that has helped European women for centuries:

European Female Tea

1 oz. cinquefoil (*Potentilla anserina*)
1 oz. camomile (*Matricaria chamomilla*)
1 oz. lady's mantle (*Alchemilla vulgaris*)
1 oz. yarrow (*Achillea millefolium*)

Use: 2 teaspoons per 1 cup hot water. Steep 10 minutes, strain, and drink 1–3 cups daily.

HOW I FLUSHED AWAY A BREAST INFECTION

Years ago, while nursing my daughter, I suddenly developed a painful breast infection. My breasts became hard; big nodules formed under the armpit, and I ran a slight fever. Nursing seemed impossible, but since I realized how important it was to stimulate the flow of milk, I did not give in to the incredible pain of nursing, but in addition, I started to pump the breasts to make sure they were emptied each time.

The whole ordeal was an incredible nightmare. I called my obstetrician and since his prognosis was most frightening, my husband and I decided to try a combination of old and new remedies first.

I mixed 20 grams (20,000 mg) of pure ascorbic acid (vitamin C) with one gallon of red grape juice and drank it all down in one day. In addition, I took 100,000 International Units of vitamin A daily, 1,000 I.U. of vitamin E daily, and a high-potency B-complex every hour. Within a day I felt noticeable relief, and the following day, I was without pain and symptom-free. All the nodules had disappeared and nursing was a joy once more. What a relief that was!

After this ordeal, I followed Mother's advice more carefully. Rule 1: Make sure breasts are regularly emptied. This helps prevent inflammation, and in addition, stimulates milk secretion. Rule 2: Drink plenty of peppermint tea (*Mentha piperita*), which promotes milk secretion, relieves nervous tension, and improves digestion. Peppermint may be considered a mild "blood cleanser."

PREVENTING MENOPAUSAL PROBLEMS

At the end of the reproductive period the ovaries gradually become inactive, reversing the changes that occurred during puberty, and while estrogen output decreases, a healthy adrenal system produces a number of sex hormones ensuring health and normal sexual function. As a result, women who have adrenal insufficiency often experience menopausal problems.

Sodium and potassium need to be properly balanced, and because a lack of estrogen decreases calcium absorption, calcium, magnesium, and vitamin D need to be supplied in adequate amounts, or deficiency symptoms such as nervousness, irritability, headaches, depression, and arthritic problems develop. A high-potency B-complex taken one to three times daily further supports the nervous system, and a daily intake of 400 to 800 I.U. of vitamin E has been known to eliminate hot flashes and night sweats.

Motherwort (*Leonurus cardiaca*) extract or wine has been used to ease menstrual problems for thousands of years. The Chinese recognized its value as did the Greeks and Romans, and today European doctors continue to endorse it for all female problems.

Motherwort Extract/Wine

Extract: Add 1–2 teaspoons fresh or dried herbs to 2 cups cold water and soak overnight. Strain and drink in mouthful doses throughout the day.

Wine: Boil 3–4 oz. of herb in 1 pint wine, and drink ½ to 1 glass per day.

OLD FOLK REMEDIES FOR PROSTATE PROBLEMS

Twenty-five percent of all men over age 52 have prostate problems, and a good number of them will eventually undergo surgery to remove the enlarged gland, which may cause agonizing symptoms of painful or difficult urination, infection, and tenderness causing sexual trauma. An increasing number of middle-aged men, however, will end up in the operating room to escape the threat of cancer.

For centuries, folk healers have promoted the use of seeds, particularly pumpkin seeds (*Cucurbita pepo or C. maxima*) to prevent and treat prostate hypertrophy and cancer with encouraging results. Investigators are convinced that chewing one handful of pumpkin seeds daily is as effective as drug treatment.

They are right, indeed. New German research indicates that pumpkin seeds contain substances that inhibit cancer growth, and as a result, an old-fashioned remedy is once more receiving much deserved attention. Pumpkin seeds are also high in zinc, protein, and fatty acid, nutrients that have been found to speed up recovery.

All infections respond well to vitamin A and C therapy, and since research indicates that infections quite possibly cause prostate enlargement, these nutrients should be supplied generously.

Dave S., a longtime patient of ours, had taken antibiotics for weeks but his prostate infection lingered. We recommended that he take a high-potency vitamin B-complex two times daily, plus 100,000 I.U. of vitamin A, 5 grams (5,000 mg) of vitamin C, and 100 mg of chelated zinc amino acid daily for two weeks. We encouraged him to eat one handful of pumpkin seeds throughout the day, and because protein helps the production of antibodies, we asked him to improve his protein intake by adding generous amounts of wheat germ, whole grains, eggs, dairy products, and soy flour to his vegetarian diet.

Dave recovered within a single week. We reduced his nutritional daily intake to 25,000 I.U. of vitamin A, 1,500 mg of vitamin C, and 50 mg of zinc chelate. His daily vitamin B-complex and protein intake was not lowered, since Dave insisted that these nutrients dramatically improved his stress tolerance. He also developed a liking for toasted pumpkin seeds, which his wife now serves mixed with nuts and sunflower seeds as a favorite snack.

****

References:

Barnes, Broda O., M.D.; Galton, Lawrence. *Hypothyroidism: The Unsuspected Illness.* Thomas Crowell, 1976.

Blaurock-Busch, E., Ph.D. *The Nutritional Management of Hypothyroidism.* Donsbach University, 1982.

Cecil-Loeb. *Textbook of Medicine.* W.B. Saunders, 1971.

Cheraskin, E., M.D., D.M.D.; Ringsdorf, W.M., Jr., D.M.D. *Predictive Medicine.* Keats, 1973.

Davis, Adelle. *Let's Get Well.* Harcourt, Brace & World, 1965.

Fredericks, Carlton, Ph.D. *New and Complete Nutrition Handbook.* Int. Institute of Natural Health Sciences, Inc., 1976.

Furlenmaier, M., M.D. *Wunderwelt der Heilpflanzen.* Zurich: Schwitter Holding AG, 1978.

Goerz, Heinz. *Gesundheit durch Heilkraeuter.* W. Moeller Verlag, 1974.

Hodges, Robert E., M.D. *Nutrition in Medical Practice.* W.B. Saunders, 1980.

Lindt, Inge. *Naturheilkunde.* Buch und Zeit Verlag, 1977.

Pfeiffer, Carl C., Ph.D., M.D. *Mental and Elemental Nutrients.* Keats Publ., 1975.

"The Prostate." *Health Express.* Vol. 2 No. 8. Nov. 1981, p. 55.

Reuben, David, M.D. *The Save Your Life Diet.* Random House, 1975.

Robinson, Corinne H. *Normal and Therapeutic Nutrition.* Macmillan, 1972.

Schauenberg, P.; Paris, F. *BLV Bestimmungsbuch.* Heilpflanzen, BLV, 1978.

Steen and Montagu. *Anatomy and Physiology.* Vol. I and II. Barnes & Noble, 1959.

Williams, Roger, J., Ph.D. *The Wonderful World Within You.* Bantam Books, 1977.

6

Achieving and Maintaining
a Healthy Nervous System

WHAT IS STRESS?

Stress and stress responses are as old as mankind. People have always faced stress, reacted to stress, and ultimately learned to protect themselves from the negative aspects of stress. While each person has his or her own stress tolerance level, which in one individual may be much higher or considerably lower than in another individual, bodily responses are similar. Stress activates the pituitary gland to secrete hormones that are transported by the blood to the adrenal glands, which respond by flooding the body with adrenalin and other stress hormones to quickly prepare the body to meet the emergency. Proteins, at first drawn from the thymus and lymph glands, are broken down to form sugars for quick energy. Blood sugar levels soar, blood pressure increases, and the individual's nutritional needs increase manyfold.

Hans Selye, world-renowned stress researcher, pointed out as early as 1938, that the body reacts to every kind of stress in the same manner, meaning that an exciting and joyful experience creates basically the same body reaction as, for instance, anxiety does. And since all stress can potentially harm the body, the demands for increased nutrition and rest must be met, or disease results. Pituitary and adrenal exhaustion can become life-threatening when exposure to stress is excessive.

IMPROVING STRESS TOLERANCE WITH EASY-TO-DO RELAXATION TECHNIQUES

Stress is a part of living; therefore, the goal is not to eliminate stress altogether (which is impossible anyway, unless you prefer the eternal alternative—death), but to improve stress tolerance. Since you cannot avoid all stressful situations it makes sense to learn how to cope with them. That's what the old folks did, and while they weren't trouble-free, their way of coping with the ups and downs of daily living compares well to modern stress seminars, which, essentially prepare you to do the same.

It's really rather simple. If your boss, spouse, friend, or children are too demanding, relax. You don't have to be Superman or Superwoman, even though you might like the idea. Admit your limits. Often, that is all it takes to receive help and understanding, and it can be a lot easier than running away from problems. Besides, running does not protect you from encountering other difficulties.

If your job is mentally draining, try "floating." It is easy to do. Lie down on the floor, or anywhere you like, and stare at the ceiling. Don't think about anything and don't try to empty your mind or concentrate. Just float. Let thoughts pass through. Don't focus. Let things happen. Your mind and body will soon achieve a deep state of relaxation that can produce astonishing results. Set aside a few minutes each day to escape the hustle and bustle of your tiresome routine, and don't think it is time wasted. It is not. These few idle minutes help you to withstand stressful situations, improve your health, and enable you to be more resourceful and productive. Try this old-fashioned stress technique that my family practiced long before stress seminars emphasized the importance of relaxation; it won't cost you more than a few minutes a day, yet the rewards are longlasting.

Is your workday too demanding and tiresome? Why not emulate Bavarian and Austrian townfolks who still recognize the importance of resting at midday. In many European countries, lunch hours are observed from noon to two. Stores close and many people go home to eat lunch, relax, even nap as their forefathers did centuries ago. Despite the twentieth century rush, there is no indication that this custom will be abandoned. My brothers are as engaged and busy as any American I know, yet their two-hour rest at midday is as sacred as ever.

You say you cannot afford such luxury? Can you afford a heart attack? Cancer? Think about it.

SIMPLE EXERCISES REDUCE MUSCLE TENSION

Listen to your body. Is there any place where you feel cramped? Does your forehead feel tense? Do your shoulders feel tight? Does your neck ache? Loosen these trouble spots with simple exercises.

1. Rotate your head in a circular motion, first to the right, then to the left. Repeat several times.
2. Roll your shoulders forward and backward several times.
3. Try to move all facial muscles by making funny faces. Open your mouth wide and stretch jaw muscles.

If you notice other tense spots take a minute to stretch and relax. If you are bound to a desk all day long, take a brief break several times during the day and get up and move. If you are on the run all day, sit down occasionally, inhale and exhale deeply, and try to calm your thoughts.

These simple exercises don't take more than two minutes, won't cost a dime, and can be done without disrupting schedules.

OLD AND NEW WAYS OF DEALING WITH MIGRAINE HEADACHES

Ten percent of the population are afflicted with migraine headaches, and 20 percent of all nonagenarians (people in their nineties) have been migraine sufferers. These statistics indicate that although migraine sufferers are frequently troubled with excruciating, disabling attacks, they are blessed with longevity. Perhaps because migraine attacks enforce rest?

Statistics also point out that migraine is twice as frequent in females and seems to run in families. Victims are generally classified as achievers and perfectionists, and in many cases, attacks start suddenly during puberty and stop when menopause is reached. A mild increase in blood pressure, commonly seen in middle-aged males or females, can also prevent migraine headaches.

Lauter Brunten, a famous physiologist of the nineteenth century, suggested that the cerebral blood vessels must be involved in migraine headaches. Today, researchers have a more in-depth explanation. "The main phenomenon observed," says Dr. Carol Schneider, of the Wardenberg Health Center in Boulder, Colorado, "is vasoconstriction. In a sense, migraines are a rebound dilation to too much vasoconstriction. And if you don't let the vasoconstriction happen, you don't get the dilation, or migraine."

Dr. Schneider, herself a migraine victim, says most migraines can be prevented with a very simple relaxation technique that has been developed by Drs. Thomas Budzynsky and Johann Stoyva of the Colorado Medical Center and is now commonly taught during biofeedback training. The technique can be learned and practiced by anyone.

According to Dr. Schneider, migraine patients generally get a warning before an attack. "Their hands get terrifically cold, sometimes as cold as 65 or 70 degrees Fahrenheit, and this low temperature signals that the constriction phase is happening."

Physiologists and psychologists agree that relaxation helps migraine sufferers to control attacks.

The relaxation technique most frequently used is simple and it is commonly referred to as temperature control training. Patients are taught to relax. Images of warmth are often employed. Think warm, patients are told. Imagine you are lying on the beach and the sun is pouring down, warming up your entire body—including your feet, legs, arms, and hands. This and similar images help the patient to raise his body temperature, thus preventing vasoconstriction and migraine headaches.

If you want to test your ability to raise your temperature, buy some temperature strips, such as the Physiological Trend Indicators by MDC in your local drugstore. Apply one of the little plastic strips to the tip of your middle finger, watch the strip change color, and compare color changes to the temperature conversion chart included in each package. When you are stressed and nervous, your temperature reading may be lower than 80 degrees Fahrenheit. Test yourself when nervous. If you can raise your temperature by 10 degrees within two minutes, you are good at instant relaxation. If you have difficulties, you had better learn how to slow down. It could mean goodbye to migraines.

Researchers at the Menninger Foundation investigated this simple biofeedback technique by leading a clinical trial involving 75 migraine sufferers. After a year or more, each patient was carefully evaluated and a marked improvement was reported in 74% of all patients.

To Dr. Schneider and many of her patients hand-warming is "a habitual thing now. Very seldom do I let my hands get cold. I practiced enough so hand-warming is a natural response now and I don't get migraine headaches. It's nice to live a stressful life without having to pay the costs."

In Germany, migraine headaches have long been treated with traditional herbal remedies and alternating hot and cold footbaths. These simple, inexpensive treatments influence blood circulation in essentially the same way as relaxation techniques—by preventing attacks by inhibiting vasoconstriction.

ALTERNATING HOT AND COLD FOOTBATHS

Fill one tub or deep pot with cold water (50 to 60 degrees Fahrenheit) and another with warm water (90 to 95 degrees Fahrenheit). Start by immersing feet into hot water for five minutes, then change to cold for 10 to 20 seconds. Repeat.

Migraine Herbal Formula 1

2 oz. peppermint (*Mentha piperita*)
1 oz. lemon balm (*Melissa off.*)
1 oz. rosmarin (*Rosmarinus off.*)
1 oz. valerian (*Valeriana off.*)

Use: Add 1–2 teaspoons of herbal mixture to 1 cup boiling-hot water. Immediately remove from heat and steep for 5–10 minutes. Strain and drink 1 cup 2 to 3 times daily.

Migraine Herbal Formula 2

2 oz. valerian (*Valeriana off.*)
2 oz. marjoram (*Origanum vulgare*)
2 oz. German camomile (*Matricaria chamomilla*)
1 oz. celandine (*Chelidonium majus*)
1 oz. fennel (*Foeniculum vulgare*)

Use: Same as above.

Low blood sugar (hypoglycemia) can cause migraine attacks. In 1963, the *New England Journal of Medicine* reported that electroencephalograms taken on 35 migraine patients during attacks showed that all patients had low blood sugar, and the lower the blood sugar, the more severe the headaches. After being placed on a high-protein, sugar-free diet, all patients experienced permanent relief.

High copper levels are also associated with migraines. When dietary zinc is supplemented, patients generally report having milder attacks that occur less frequently.

RELIEVING STRESS WITH FOOD AND NUTRITIONAL SUPPLEMENTS

Stress reactions do not have to be devastating. By changing habits and environment, certain stressors can be avoided, and when this is not feasible, rest and nutrition are the best and most logical preventive measures.

Medical studies demonstrate that exposure to emotional or physical stress tremendously increases the body's nutritional needs for protein; linoleic acid; the vitamins A, C and E; all the B-vitamins; and minerals such as zinc. If, for instance, protein is supplied inadequately, thymus and lymph gland tissue are harmed and the body becomes even less resistant to disease.

"Studies with animals have demonstrated that the ascorbic acid (vitamin C) content of the adrenal glands decreases when animals are stressed," Dr. Carl C. Pfeiffer of the Brain Bio Center comments, which causes animals to produce massive quantities of vitamin C. If translated into human terms, the human requirement for vitamin C during stressful situations may exceed 10 grams per day.

Human studies further indicate that vitamin C is needed to combat stress because this vitamin helps to detoxify harmful substances that are produced in greater amounts during stress. Psychiatric patients, for instance, are highly stressed individuals with unusually high demands for vitamin C and other nutrients. If these individual nutritional needs are met, improvement is usually dramatic.

Vitamin E is needed for proper function of the pituitary gland and prevents hormones from being destroyed by oxygen. The B-vitamins, commonly called the "stress vitamins," are instrumental to the proper functioning of the nervous system, and if given in large amounts, they can greatly improve stress symptoms such as depression, anxiety, insomnia. Calcium helps regulate the sympathetic nervous system and is required for muscle relaxation and contraction. It assists in sustaining heart rate and intestinal contractions in conjunction with the vitamin B-complex.

A few years back, British, Canadian, and U.S. investigators related evidence correlating soft water with heart disease. They found that heart attacks are 20 to 30 percent more frequent among people who consume soft water. Calcium and magnesium contents control water hardness: the more of the two minerals, the harder the water. Calcium is also acted upon by the thyroid as thyro-calcitonin, a substance which decreases blood calcium concentration and inhibits bone breakdown. During infections and all stress, calcium is utilized rapidly for repair of tissues in conjunction with magnesium; unsaturated fatty acids; and the vitamins A, C, and pantothenic acid. If you don't get enough calcium from your diet, consider taking a properly balanced supplement.

THE ANTISTRESS DIET PROGRAM

Breakfast:

fresh fruit or juice

1 or 2 eggs, sprinkled with wheat germ

sprouts

whole grain bread

butter

raw honey or homemade jam (should be avoided by hypoglycemic patients)

peppermint or rosehip tea, coffee-substitute, or milk

Supplements:

Take 1 teaspoon hypoallergenic amino acids 20 minutes before breakfast

With meal take: High-potency B-complex

multivitamin and mineral supplement containing 25,000 I.U. of vitamin A

1 tablespoon granulated lecithin

2 dolomite or bonemeal tablets or other calcium-magnesium product

1–2 adrenal extract tablet

1,500 mg vitamin C

Mid-Morning Snack:

1 cup unsweetened yogurt with fresh fruit, sprinkled with wheat germ, or

1 cup unsweetened whole grain cereal with milk and extra wheat germ, or

1 cup raw carrots, celery, or other vegetable

Supplements:

1 high-potency B-complex

400 I.U. of vitamin E

Lunch:

> 1 serving meat (preferably liver or lamb), fish or fowl
>
> 1 serving beets
>
> 1 serving of salad with vinegar and oil dressing (use sunflower or safflower oil), or yogurt or buttermilk dressing
>
> fruit
>
> 1 cup lemon balm tea
>
> *or*
>
> 1 cup of homemade borscht
>
> whole grain bread with tuna salad
>
> fresh vegetables
>
> fruit
>
> lemon balm tea
>
> *or*
>
> 1 cup homemade borscht
>
> 1 omelet
>
> 1 serving of salad with homemade dressing
>
> fruit
>
> lemon balm tea

> *Supplements:*
>
> Take 1 teaspoon hypoallergenic amino acid 20 minutes before meal
>
> With meal take: 1 high-potency B-complex
>
> 1,500 mg of vitamin C
>
> 2 dolomite or bonemeal tablets or other calcium-magnesium product
>
> 150 mg of zinc amino acid chelate (= .15 mg of elemental zinc), depending on need
>
> 100 mg RNA/DNA
>
> 2 multiglandular extracts

Mid-Afternoon Snack:

> ½ cup raw almonds
>
> 1 apple
>
> rosehip, peppermint or camomile tea, or milk

Supplements:

1,500 mg of vitamin C

1 high-potency B-complex

1 lymph extract

Dinner:

Same as lunch, except smaller portions. Should be a light meal.

Supplements:

1 high-potency B-complex

2 dolomite or bonemeal tablets or other calcium-magnesium product

2 cups acidophilus milk, unless yogurt is part of the daily diet

lemon balm or hop tea

Bedtime Snack:

1 bran wafer or whole wheat crackers and/or cheese

1 cup warm milk, or hop or lemon balm herb tea

ANCIENT HERBAL REMEDIES STRENGTHEN YOUR NERVOUS SYSTEM

St. Johnswort (*Hypericum perforatum*) has long been prescribed for the treatment of nervous ailments. Hippocrates and other physicians of ancient Greece used this medicinal herb as did many great healers of the Middle Ages. Today, European doctors continue to employ this medicinal herb to strengthen the nervous system. St. Johnswort, European researchers say, improves concentration; helps eliminate depression, headaches, dizziness, and insomnia; and has been successfully used among patients who have suffered nerve damage.

The Romans were fond of lavender (*Lavandula angustifolia*) and used its extract as a relaxing bath additive. Paracelsus, Kneipp, and other European folk healers equally appreciated its medicinal value for its calming properties, which aid nervous heart ailments, insomnia, dizziness, migraines, and neuralgia.

Lemon balm (*Melissa officinalis*) gained popularity during the Middle Ages. Monks brought this lemony-tasting spice to European monastery gardens and eventually discovered and made use of its healing properties. In 1611, members of the Parisian Carmelite Order introduced lemon balm tincture as "Carmelite Spirit," to the French public. This natural remedy was and continues to be recommended as an effective internal and external treatment for all nervous ailments. Today, "Carmelite Spirit" and various other brands continue to be sold in European drugstores and apothecaries. Recent European pharmaceutical studies indicate that, indeed, lemon balm tincture relaxes and strengthens the nervous system.

Modified "Carmelite Spirit"

4 oz. lemon balm leaves, crushed
2 oz. lemon peel, cut
1 oz. nutmeg, ground
½ oz. cinnamon, ground
½ oz. cloves, ground
8 oz. of 70% alcohol

Combine all ingredients, pour into bottle and store in a dark, cool area. Let mixture steep for two weeks, but shake once or twice daily. Strain into clean bottle and use internally, 1–2 teaspoons daily with water. Children: 10–15 drops daily with water. "Carmelite spirit" can also be used as a rub for arthritic pain, headaches, and migraines.

Herbal Stress-Fighter

Strengthens and calms the nervous system; useful for neurasthenia, anxiety.)

1 oz. St. Johnswort (*Hypericum perforatum*)
1 oz. lavender (*Lavandula officinalis*)
2 oz. lemon balm (*Melissa officinalis*)

Use: Add 1 teaspoon to 1 cup boiling-hot water. Remove from heat immediately and steep for 3–5 minutes. Strain and drink 1–3 cups per day.

CLASSICAL TREATMENTS FOR HYPERTENSION

Any form of stress can increase hypertension, and if you already suffer from elevated blood pressure, improving your stress resistance is important. Learn to slow down, eat the best diet possible, and reduce salt (sodium) intake to a minimum. If you are overweight, start a sensible weight loss program *today*.

Be kind to your kidneys, whose function is to control blood pressure. When the kidneys are damaged, blood pressure often increases dramatically.

Start walking. European doctors have recommended this simple exercise in the treatment of hypertension with excellent results. Spa treatments do not only enforce hydrotherapy and a sensible diet; equal attention is paid to proper exercise and walking, which, spa doctors say, is still the simplest and most sensible exercise of all. A brisk half-hour walk each day can do wonders for your blood pressure.

Avoid alcohol, coffee, nicotine, and all other stimulants, but drink plenty of herb teas to support kidney function (see Chapter 4). Ask your nutritionist or nutritionally-oriented doctor for a mineral hair analysis and have him evaluate possible toxic minerals in your system, because cadmium, in particular, is associated with high blood pressure and kidney failure. Avoid all possible sources of cadmium contamination such as leaking batteries, cadmium vapor lamps, water, coffee, tea (not herbal tea), cigarette smoke, and hobbies using solders. If your cadmium level is high, take a zinc supplement. Zinc antagonizes cadmium.

HERBS THAT REGULATE BLOOD PRESSURE

Garlic (*Allium sativum*), is considered an important biocatalyst by European phytotherapists, because it activates biological processes. Known for centuries as an invaluable medicine, garlic has proven useful in the treatment of numerous diseases including infections and digestive and respiratory ailments. European research indicates that garlic effectively lowers high blood pressure and counteracts arteriosclerosis.

Use: ½ teaspoon garlic oil (3–6 capsules) per day.

Hawthorn flowers (*Crataegus oxyacantha*) slowly regulate blood pressure, and improve all nervous and degenerative heart problems without causing side effects.

Use: 1–2 teaspoons per 1 cup hot water. Steep 10 minutes, strain, and drink 1 cup 2–3 times daily.

Onion (*Allium cepa*). Ancient China and Egypt recognized this vegetable for its excellent medicinal properties. Similar in action, but somewhat less effective than garlic oil, onion juice is known to lower blood pressure and regenerate health. European health care providers recommend it for neuralgias.

Use: 1–3 tablespoons onion juice per day (unless intake causes gastric disturbances, which may indicate a food sensitivity).

Mistletoe (*Viscum album*). This medicinal herb has been highly regarded among European health care providers since ancient times, and continues to be widely used among modern European physicians. Since the FDA restricted its use, this medicinal herb is not easily available to the American consumer, largely because mistletoe, if used in *extremely* high doses, can induce cardiac arrest. Modern research indicates, however, that *small* doses of this semiparasitic herb *strengthen* cardiac function and act as a vasodilator, thus lowering blood pressure. In addition, European scientists recently isolated a protein from this herb that has been found to inhibit cancer growth in animals.

Use: Add 2–3 teaspoons herb to 1 cup cold water. Let soak overnight, strain, and drink 1–3 cups before meals.

Note: European drugstores carry a wide variety of mistletoe preparations that often contain hawthorn and garlic, and these herbal remedies are widely recommended and prescribed by medical doctors.

As a columnist for *Bestways* magazine, I can count on enlightened readers' responses. Lisa R.'s letter was especially heartwarming. She wrote:

Dear Eleonore:
My husband has been on blood pressure medication for twenty-three years. It controlled his blood pressure but over the last few years he seemed to develop kidney problems. When I read your article about herbs that control blood pressure I decided to give it a try. I put him on garlic (eight capsules a day) and through a German friend, I bought several packages of a mistletoe-hawthorn preparation. To make a long story short, my husband is now off his blood pressure medication but continues to take garlic and the German mistletoe preparation, which I now buy through a Chicago drugstore. He really feels so much better now. We are very grateful for your help. God bless you.

OLD-FASHIONED CALMATIVES AND SEDATIVES

Herbal calmatives and/or sedatives are preferred to drugs by many European health care providers who prescribe them for a number of nervous ailments, including tension headaches, anxiety, nervous heart problems, hypertension, and insomnia. The medicinal herbs listed below have a tranquilizing effect and are not addictive.

Hops (*Humulus lupulus*) are a mild sedative. Reduces anxiety, nervousness, restlessness, insomnia.

Use: 1–2 teaspoons hops per 1 cup hot water. Cover and steep 10 minutes. Strain and drink warm, 1 cup before bedtime. Hops should be used fresh, because storage reduces effectiveness.

Passion flower (*Passiflora incarnata*) is a strong sedative and antispasmodic. Good for all nervous conditions, including insomnia, restlessness, tension headaches, and migraines. Use professional preparations only. Passion flower is often found in herbal sedatives.

Valerian root (*Valeriana officinalis*) is a calmative and antispasmodic. Influences the central nervous system. Recommended for all nervous problems. Especially useful for patients suffering from stress symptoms such as tension headaches, spastic conditions, and digestive problems due to nervousness. Induces sleep.

Use: Add 2–3 teaspoons valerian root to 2 cups cold water. Heat up, but do not boil, and let soak for several hours. Strain and drink in small doses throughout the day. To induce sleep, drink 1 cup after dinner and another before retiring.

OVERCOMING INSOMNIA WITH TRADITIONAL HERBAL NIGHTCAPS

Mild

2 oz. camomile (*Matricaria chamomilla*)
2 oz. hops (*Humulus lupulus*)
1 oz. anise seed (*Pimpinella anisum*)
1 oz. dill seed (*Anethum graveolens*)

Use: Add 1 teaspoon of herbal mixture to 1 cup boiling-hot water. Immediately remove from heat and steep for 3–5 minutes. (Longer steeping can cause bitter taste.) Drink 1–2 cups warm before bedtime. Good for children.

Moderate Strength

1 oz. hops (*Humulus lupulus*)
1 oz. lemon balm (*Melissa off.*)
2 oz. valerian root (*Valeriana off.*)

Use: Add 1 teaspoon of herbal mixture to 1 cup cold water. Heat up, but do not boil. Remove from heat and steep for one or more hours. Strain and drink 1–2 cups before bedtime.

Strong

2 oz. valerian root (*Valeriana off.*)
1 oz. lemon balm leaves (*Melissa off.*)
1 oz. lavender flowers (*Lavandula off.*)
1 oz. passion flower (*Passiflora incarnata*). Do not use more!

Use: Add 1 teaspoon herbal mixture to 1 cup hot water, steep for 10 minutes, strain, and drink warm, 1½ to 1 cup before bedtime, depending on age.

GRANDMA'S SIMPLE TREATMENT FOR INSOMNIA

Benjamin Franklin frequently suffered from sleeplessness, and his remedy for this was rather odd. Since he believed that a warm bed caused him to wake up prematurely, he kept two beds, just in case. When he woke up at night, something that happened quite often, he moved from the warm bed to the cold one. He really should have had a cup of milk.

Warm milk with honey was my maternal grandmother's old-fashioned insomnia treatment and it worked everytime. Why? Milk contains tryptophan, which scientists say is an amino acid essential for proper metabolic function. Tryptophan is a precursor of niacin and the neurotransmitter serotin. Researchers believe that serotin and sleep are intimately related.

Unlike a sleeping pill, tryptophan does not change the insomniac's sleeping pattern. On the contrary, it induces a natural sleep without causing after-effects such as morning drowsiness. Foods high in tryptophan are milk, all other dairy products, and meat. Since turkey is especially high in tryptophan, insomnia should be less of a problem Thanksgiving night.

THERAPEUTIC BATHING FOR A HEALTHY NERVOUS SYSTEM

"The piping hot bath," Dr. Carl Pfeiffer writes, "has biophysical logic. Muscle when tense, is in high state of tone. Heat forces the muscle into relaxed submission." In simple terms, too much muscle tightness, or tone, constricts blood vessels, causing a decrease in blood flow. Heat dilates blood vessels, thus it promotes and improves blood circulation.

Orientals have made use of this principle for centuries. In Japan business meetings are often held in large, steaming community tubs where relaxation comes naturally. In Europe therapeutic bathing combines three natural healers: herbs, heat, and water.

While most people enjoy relaxing in a steaming hot tub, old and very young people often feel uncomfortable in a hot bath (over 100 degrees Fahrenheit). Since high temperatures can shock the system and cause increased heart action, hot baths are not recommended for people suffering from nervous heart ailments, hypertension, and similar nervous problems.

Warm baths (90 to 95 degrees Fahrenheit) relax and calm the nervous system. Add the proper herbs and you can have your own spa treatment in the privacy of your own home. It's an inexpensive, healthy luxury nobody should do without.

Bath Additives

1. Relaxing, calming—for nervous tension, hypertension, insomnia

Camomile flowers (*Matricaria chamomilla*)
Hops (*Humulus lupulus*)
Lavender (*Lavandula off.*)
Lemon balm (*Melissa off.*)
Oat straw (*Avena sativa*)
Thyme (*Thymus vulgaris*)
Valerian (*Valeriana off.*)

2. Stimulating—improves energy

Birch leaves (*Betula alba*)
Juniper twigs (*Juniperus communis*)
Pine twigs or young green cones (*Picea excelsa*)
Rosmarin (*Rosmarinus off.*)
Sweet flag rootstock (*Acorus calamus*)

Use sufficient water to cover 1 lb. of herb, bring to boil, steep 10–30 minutes, strain, and add to tub water. Add strained herb into linen cloth, and hang cloth into bath water for additional extraction.

REDUCING NIGHT SWEATING—NATURALLY

Night sweats are commonly associated with the menopause, and while women are more frequently afflicted with this problem, people of both sexes and all ages may experience this discomforting problem. Nutritional reports indicate that night sweats due to the menopause often disappear when 100 to 600 I.U. of vitamin E is taken daily, but quickly recur when the vitamin is stopped.

While attending the Seventeenth Convention of the German Association for Osteopathy and Chiropractic (ACO), held in 1977 in Bad Kissingen, I mentioned to Health Practitioner Schumacher that my daughter, then four years old, often woke up in the middle of the night bathed in sweat. A few weeks later, I received a small package containing a homeopathic remedy containing calcium carbonate. According to instructions, three of the tiny tablets were to be taken daily until all symptoms disappeared.

Honestly, I was somewhat skeptical that these minute amounts of calcium carbonate would make a difference, but soon, the night sweats recurred less frequently, and within a month disappeared altogether.

German and other European health care providers often recommend herbal teas to reduce night sweating. Wild strawberry leaves (*Fragria vesca*), walnut leaves (*Juglans regia*), tormentil rootstock (*Potentilla erecta*), hops (*Humulus lupulus*), hyssop (*Hyssopus officinalis*), lemon balm

(*Melissa officinalis*), sage (*Salvia officinalis*), and stinging nettle leaves (*Urtica dioica*) all have been found to benefit patients suffering from recurring night sweating.

The following herbal tea mixture reduces perspiration and night sweats. Its main ingredient, sage, effectively inhibits sweat gland activity, thus this remedy should be taken only temporarily and not be given to children.

Herbal Formula to Reduce Nervous Perspiration and Night Sweats

> 2 oz. sage (*Salvia off.*)
> 1 oz. walnut leaves (*Juglans regia*)
> 1 oz. hyssop (*Hyssopus officinalis*)
> 1 oz. stinging nettle leaves (*Urtica dioica*)
> Use: Steep 2 teaspoons of herbal mixture in ½ cup boiling-hot water for 10 minutes. Strain and drink in small doses throughout the day to stop excess perspiration. To prevent night sweating, drink ½ cup before bedtime.

DIET AS PART OF ALCOHOLIC'S RECOVERY PROGRAM

Alcoholism is a serious disease and few patients are more in need of nutritional care than the chronic alcoholic.

The very first thing alcoholics must do is *stop drinking completely*. After this they need to take steps to rebuild their shattered health, and here improved nutrition can play an important role.

"Nutritional deficiencies constitute a major part of the alcoholic patient's ills,"[1] says Dr. Robert Hodges, Professor of Internal Medicine at the California School of Medicine. Alcohol may seem like food to the alcoholic, but its nutritional value is ridiculously inadequate. As a result, chronic alcoholics are generally severely deficient in most nutrients, particularly thiamin, ascorbic acid, folates, niacin, iron magnesium, zinc, and others. Since alcohol acts as a diuretic, water-soluble nutrients are readily lost via the urine.

Researchers such as Drs. Cheraskin, Roger Williams, and others have noted repeatedly that when all needed nutrients are sufficiently supplied, patients report a reduced craving for alcohol, and their formerly grossly inadequate dietary habits improve, as do related health problems

---

[1]Used with permission of W.B. Saunders Publ. Co. From *Nutrition in Medical Practice*, by Robert E. Hodges, M.D.

such as hypertension, high cholesterol and triglyceride levels, digestive problems, liver disease, or dermatitis.

A highly nutritious diet supplying adequate protein should be part of the alcoholic's recovery program. Glandular extracts such as liver extract support this stressed gland and should be part of this program along with vitamin C and other nutrients. Adequate vitamin C intake, Dr. G. Milner, Registrar of Psychiatry at the Towers Hospital in Leicester, England, reports, markedly improves states of depression and anxiety which are psychiatric disorders commonly found among alcoholics. German health care providers also recommend beet juice or milk thistle tea to improve liver function, and small doses of birch leaf juice or tea to strengthen kidney and bladder function (see Chapter 4).

HERBAL STIMULANTS

The mild herbal stimulants included here improve circulation and influence the nervous system. Unlike narcotics, which at first greatly increase vital activity, and later cause exhaustion, the following old-fashioned herbal formulas have tonic properties and increase nervous activity only slightly. Ginseng (*Panax quinquefolius* or *P. schinseng*), for years has been considered a panacea for all ailments, and is an excellent tonic and stimulant that benefits people of all ages. Drink one to three cups per day to improve energy and well-being.

Formula 1

1 oz. blackberry leaves (*Rubus villosus*)
1 oz. raspberry leaves (*Rubus idaeus or R. strigosus*)
1 oz. wild hyssop (*Pycnanthemum virginianum*)
1 oz. yarrow (*Achillea millefolium*)

Formula 2

1 oz. cardamom (*Elettaria cardomomum*)
1 oz. ginger (*Zingiber officinale*)
1 oz. lemon balm (*Melissa off.*)
2 oz. raspberry leaves (*Rubus idaeus or R. strigosus*)

Use: Add 1 teaspoon of herbal mixture to 1 cup boiling-hot water. Steep 5 minutes, strain and drink, one or more cups per day.

****

References:

Cheraskin, E., M.D.; Ringsdorf, W.M., D.M.D.; Clark, J.W., D.D.S. *Diet and Disease.* Keats, 1968.

Davis, Adelle. *Let's Get Well.* Harcourt, Brace and World, 1965.

Executive Health. Vol. XIV, 2, Nov. 1977.

Fredericks, Carlton, Ph.D. *New & Complete Nutrition Handbook.* Major Books, 1974.

Furlenmeier, M., M.D. *Wunderwelt der Heilpflanzen.* Schwitter Holding AG, 1978.

Goerz, Heinz. *Gesundheit durch Heilkraeuter.* W. Moeller Verlag, 1974.

Grieve, M. *A Modern Herbal.* Dover, 1971.

Heinerman, John. *Science of Herbal Medicine.* By-World, 1979.

Hodges, Robert E., M.D. *Nutrition in Medical Practice.* Saunders, 1980.

Hutchens, Alma R. *Indian Herbology of North America.* Merco, 1973.

Lindt, Inge. *Naturheilkunde.* Buch und Zeit Verlagsges., 1977.

Lamott. "What to Do When Stress Signs Say You're Killing Yourself." *Today's Health,* Jan. 1975.

Lust, John. B., N.D., D.B.M. *The Herb Book.* Bantam, 1974.

Pfeiffer, Carl C. *Mental and Elemental Nutrients.* Keats Publ., 1975.

Robinson, Corinne, H., M.S., R.D. *Normal and Therapeutic Nutrition.* Macmillan, 1972.

Schauenberg, P.; Paris, F. *BLV Bestimmungsbuch.* BLV Verlag, 1978.

Stage, Wolfgang, M.D. *Das Kneipp Taschenbuch.* Ullstein, 1968.

Steen, Edwin B.; Montagu, Ashley, Ph.D.s. *Anatomy and Physiology.* Vol. 2. Barnes and Noble, 1959.

7

Old-Country Remedies Add Youthfulness to Skin, Hair and Nails

BEAUTY STARTS WITHIN

Glowing skin, shiny hair, and healthy nails have always been considered keynotes of beauty, and while heredity decides whether you are fair-skinned and freckled, naturally blond, or black-haired with dark complexion, your health determines how beautiful your exterior really is.

The main organs involved in the elimination process are the colon, liver, kidney, and the skin, which covers approximately nineteen square feet and weighs about seven pounds. Since the skin eliminates approximately twenty percent of the body's toxic waste, excess waste is stressful to the skin, resulting in skin problems. Though some dermatologists feel that diet does not play an important part in the treatment of skin disorders, nutritionally-oriented doctors generally believe that it does. Or, as Mother continues to tell anyone willing to listen, "You are what you eat," and "cleanliness is health and beauty."

When nutrition and hygiene are less than adequate, the skin, hair, and nails suffer and all the attractively packaged cosmetics in the world won't help. Just read the labels of those elegant looking and smelling facial creams. Isn't it astonishing how many chemicals are packed into these fine beauty products? Can they really be good for you?

TREATING ACNE, MOTHER'S WAY

"Acne," a German doctor once said, "is one of the diseases that won't kill you, but it can ruin your life." Unlike my brother, I never suffered from ugly acne problems because I tried to follow Mother's advice. Her treatment plan was simple but rigid and included many dos and do nots, though the reward—healthy, glowing skin—was worth every effort.

Do not: smoke; drink alcohol, coffee, tea (except herbals); take drugs, unless your doctor tells you to; eat foods that constipate you; eat animal fats and food prepared in cheap cooking oil; eat sugary foods including chocolate; take chemical laxatives; use perfumed soaps, facial creams, and make up; do not treat affected area with alcoholic cleansers.

Do: eat plenty of fresh fruit and raw vegetables, particularly carrots, celery, lettuce, sprouts, and watercress; eat steamed beets or drink ½ cup of beet juice once or twice weekly; take 2–3 tablespoons of wheat germ daily; take 2–3 tablespoons of Brewer's yeast daily; eat whole grain bread only; eat plenty of plain yogurt; drink 2 cups buttermilk per day.

To satisfy your "sweet tooth," eat dried apricots, figs, and dates; eat 1 to 2 tablespoons of linseed (*Linum usitatissimum*); reduce salt intake to minimum; use safflower, soy, or sunflower oil for cooking. Use a pH-controlled soap; use camomile vapor bath three times per week to soften and cleanse skin. Use witch hazel decoction for further cleansing. Do not use any commercial facial creams or lotions, use fresh aloe vera juice, instead. Apply to freshly cleansed skin three times daily. If skin feels too dry apply wheat germ oil.

Once weekly, apply fresh savoy leaves to affected area followed by rinse with camomile or witch hazel decoction; start nine-day blood cleansing program.

OLD-TIME BLOOD CLEANSE

Anybody interested in health and beauty should use this blood cleansing program two to four times per year. Fasting is not required but the juices should be taken ½ hour before meals and should always be diluted with six times the amount of water. You can either juice fresh herbs or use commercial brands as found in health food stores.

1. To the third day: take two tablespoons nettle juice (*Urtica dioica*) mornings and one tablespoon before lunch and dinner.
2. To sixth day: use same amount of dandelion juice.
3. To ninth day: use same amount of celery juice.

Mother recommended this treatment to many young friends and customers, but the most dramatic recovery was made by an apprentice who was troubled with an extreme case of acne. The young lady had been to several dermatologists with no results, and though she was on the verge of giving up, Mother persuaded her to give it another try. Irene did, but after four weeks she was still discouraged and depressed because "the miracle just won't happen." Mother had another talk with Irene who then continued the program. Six months later, her skin finally cleared. Mother's reaction? "I told you so!" By the way, Irene, who once was shy and intimidated, turned into an outgoing, fun-loving lady and became a wonderful friend.

CUSTOMARY EUROPEAN SKIN TREATMENTS

Europeans are known to use a variety of fruits, herbs, and vegetables to aid the skin with excellent results. As a matter of fact, these old-fashioned beauty and health treatments are more effective than the majority of modern cosmetics, which, most often, camouflage skin conditions instead of improving them. Not infrequently, the application of artificially flavored and colored lotions of mineral oil basis to trouble spots only worsens the problem.

Fresh, organic savory leaves, applied to the skin, absorb toxins, thus preventing and healing troublesome skin problems.

Use clean, fresh leaves only. Remove the hard inner core and, with a rolling-pin, try flattening them like pizza dough. Hold leaves over steam and apply warm to affected area. Change when cold, but never use the same leaf twice. After the treatment gently massage wheat germ oil into skin. Treat your skin to this procedure once daily for one to two weeks until an improvement is apparent.

Strawberry facials clean pores, nourish the skin, and help clear up adolescent acne and similar skin problems. Simply mash fresh strawberries and spread the pretty pink paste all over your face, but do not cover eyes. Leave on for 10 to 15 minutes and rinse off with cold water.

OLD-FASHIONED TREATMENT FOR SKIN INFECTIONS

The overall treatment is similar to the acne program, though the blood cleanse should continue for two weeks. One-half to one cup of carrot juice diluted with six times the amount of water should be taken from the tenth to the fourteenth day. In addition, 400 I.U. of vitamin E and 15 mg or more of zinc are to be taken daily for a minimum of three months to improve healing.

Shave grass (*Equisetum arvense*) hot packs have been recommended for dry skin infections by European folk healers for centuries. Sebastian Kneipp was especially fond of these remedies and used them extensively in the treatment of skin ailments. Add one handful or more of the herb to cold water and bring to boil. Simmer for three minutes, strain, and spread herb on clean cloth. Wrap and apply to affected area. Leave on until cold, and wash skin well with camomile (*Matricaria chamomilla*) infusion. Use once daily.

When large areas are affected, shave grass can be used as a bath additive. Add one pound shave grass to one quart water, bring to boil, and simmer for 5 to 10 minutes. Strain, wrap herb into linen cloth, and hang into tub water. Add decoction to tub water and bathe for 10 to 15 minutes. If skin feels dry, apply wheat germ oil.

If the problem skin blisters and wets, apply the following herbal poultice:

Herbal Poultice for Skin Infections

Mix equal amounts of camomile flowers (*Matricaria chamomilla*), wheat germ, bran, and crushed oat straw. Add sufficient hot water to form a thick paste, wrap in thin linen cloth, and apply to affected area. Leave on for 10 minutes or more, remove and wash skin with camomile infusion or soak in shave grass or camomile bath.

ANCIENT MUD TREATMENTS HELP ECZEMAS AND RASHES

Anthropological studies suggest that mud treatments have been used since antiquity and may be as old as man himself. In ancient societies, mud spas became the Mecca of the ill, for mud heals infections, skin ulcers, and swollen tissues. Today, European, particularly Russian, mud spas are still thriving. Respected, knowledgeable physicians prescribe mud therapy to ailing people of all ages, and health insurance agents have no complaints about it. In Europe, mud treatments are considered common medical treatments.

The healing power of mud has puzzled medical people for centuries and initiated numerous speculations and theories that tried to explain the healing properties of mud. During the Middle Ages people believed that ghosts and spirits which supposedly were housed in the soft wet earth were responsible for miraculous healings, though more scientific minds speculated that the warmth alone alleviated ailments. Others thought that the simple yet strong belief in the curative power of mud accounted for amazing recoveries and cures.

Modern researchers know better. According to Professor Stoeber of the Austrian Institute of Mud Research (yes, this and other such respected institutions exist throughout Europe), heat is not as important to mud treatments as formerly thought, because mud also heals when applied cold. Its function, Professor Stoeber says, is strictly biochemical. For one thing, not all mud has healing properties. The type of mud that does is mildly acidic with a pH slightly below 7. Scientists have demonstrated that in this environment, microorganisms such as penicillin, streptomyces, and actinomyces thrive.

In addition, healing mud is rich in certain minerals and contains high amounts of unsaturated fatty acids such as linoleic, linolenic and arachidonic acids—all essential to proper skin care. As Professor Stoeber points out, the biochemical action of healing mud is rather complex. Though it mainly detoxifies the skin, healing mud also influences the nervous system and certain organs. Therefore, mud baths are not recommended for those suffering from acute genital infections, emphysema, heart problems, or tuberculosis. Pregnant women should also avoid mud treatments.

Russian and other European mud research indicate that mud baths, mud packs, and similar treatments are extremely valuable for skin ulcers, eczemas, and other skin conditions and may be considered superior to drug treatment.

Therefore, if you have an unsolved skin problem, get some dry mud from your local health food store and use it according to directions. You will be in for a pleasant surprise. Also, since mud packs dry out the skin, use wheat germ oil, peanut oil, or walnut oil to soften your skin.

Interestingly, nutritional studies indicate that those individuals afflicted with psoriasis, an eczema-like skin condition, are generally deficient in the vitamins A and B6 and lecithin, and when these nutrients are supplied improvement is evident.

STEAMING AWAY UGLY BOILS

To make a facial steam bath you need a chair, a pot that holds about a gallon of water, some towels, and the herbs camomile and yarrow, also called milfoil (*Achillea millefolium*).

Bring water to a quick boil, add ½ cup each of camomile and yarrow flowers, and quickly reduce heat. Arrange a chair so that you can hold your head comfortably over the pot to steam your face. Drape the towels around your head and the pot and let the herbal vapors penetrate your skin as long as it feels comfortable.

Have a pot of witch hazel (*Hamamelis virginiana*) infusion ready to be used as a skin cleanser. To make it, boil three tablespoons witch hazel bark or leaves in one pint water for three to five minutes and strain. After the steam treatment, wet a cotton ball or facial tissue with witch hazel infusion and thoroughly cleanse skin. If the boils are ready to be opened, use two facial tissues and gently squeeze open, but do not use fingernails. Clean again with witch hazel decoction and rub zinc ointment onto affected area.

GERMAN REMEDY FOR ITCHING SKIN PROBLEMS

In my family, bran treatments are still recommended for itching skin problems, an old-time remedy known and employed by German health practitioner Leipold of Karlsruhe says, decrease itching and promote healing. To make a bran poultice, add sufficient hot water to bran to form a paste and spread over affected area. After it has dried, wash away with lukewarm water followed by cold rinse. (Alternating warm and cold showers stimulates circulation and stimulates needed elimination of toxins.) Prepare arnica decoction, soak cotton ball or facial tissue, and gently cleanse skin. Prepare Iceland moss infusion and drink one cup per day for four weeks, or more.

Arnica Cleanse

(*for external use*)

Add 2 heaping teaspoons of arnica flowers (*Arnica montana*) to 1 cup boiling water and steep for 5 to 10 minutes. Strain or filter, using paper filter.

Iceland Moss Decoction

(*for internal use*)

Add 2 tablespoons of Iceland moss (*Cetraria islandica*) to 1 cup boiling-hot water and boil for 10 minutes. Strain and drink.

EUROPEAN FOLK REMEDY FOR SKIN ULCERS

Since all skin ailments start from within, European holistic doctors like the German Dr. Otto F. Buchinger and the Swiss Dr. Ralph Bircher recommend first of all that patients suffering from skin ulcers start on a juice fast, followed by a salt-free vegetarian diet consisting of raw fruits and vegetables. Fenugreek (*Trigonella foenum-graecum*) poultices are to be applied daily followed with warm and cold camomile compresses and the

Arnica Cleanse (see section on "German Remedy for Itching Skin Problems").

Vegetable Juice Fast

Juices provide excellent nourishment as they are loaded with vitamins and minerals. Combining various fruit and vegetable juices, or the addition of lime or lemon juice, helps improve nutritional value, flavor and taste.

Previous to your juice fast, take a mild herbal laxative with plenty of water. Use a variety of juices such as carrot, celery, and tomato juice, including 1 cup of sauerkraut juice per day, and dilute them fifty-fifty with plain water or mineral water. Vegetable broth and herb teas such as peppermint, rosehips and others can be taken between juices. Your total liquid intake should be a minimum of 8 glasses.

Your fast should not continue for more than 8 days, and should *be supervised by a qualified health care provider.* After you decide to break your fast, start eating small meals. Even if food looks tempting, Do Not Overeat.

Fenugreek Poultice

Add sufficient hot water and 1 teaspoon apple cider vinegar to 4 tablespoons powdered fenugreek seeds and 4 tablespoons powdered fenugreek root to form paste. Apply to ulcer and leave on for ½ hour or more. Rinse off with lukewarm water, followed by cold rinse and apply alternating warm and cold camomile compresses.

Camomile Compress

Add 1 tablespoon camomile flowers (*Matricaria chamomilla*) to 1–2 cups hot water. Remove from heat, steep for 5 minutes, strain or filter. Soak clean cloth or towel in this infusion, wring out excess, and apply to affected area. Cover with dry towel and leave on for 15 to 20 minutes. Remove and clean area with arnica cleanse.

INDIAN REMEDY FOR CANCEROUS SKIN ULCERS

The Indians used pokeweed (*Phytolacca americana*) poultices made from dried powdered leaves or roots to alleviate all sorts of skin ailments including inflammations, swellings, and cancerous skin ulcers. Fresh leaf poultices applied to old scabs were used to speed up the healing process with good results.

Early settlers used pokeweed berry juice to treat skin eruptions and cancerous skin ulcers. New research substantiates that pokeweed berries inhibit the division of body cells, a basic requirement for the treatment of tumors and cancers. *The berries, however, should NOT be eaten. Their seeds are poisonous.*

Pokeweed Poultice

To make a pokeweed poultice add sufficient water to powdered, dried pokeweed leaves or roots to form paste. Apply to affected area and cover with clean cloth. Remove poultice after 10 to 20 minutes and cleanse skin with camomile decoction.

PREVENTING SCAR TISSUES AND STRETCH MARKS

Nutritionists often promote the use of vitamin E for the prevention and treatment of stretch marks and scar tissue, and though various sources report varying results, I am positive that vitamin E, if used properly, can improve and even restore weakened skin tissue.

After my firstborn, I developed ugly stretch marks along the upper part of my legs and when I was expecting again (eight years later at the age of 32) I immediately increased my vitamin E intake to 600 International Units and started applying vitamin E oil to those trouble spots. I also took a high-potency vitamin B complex; a multivitamin supplement containing 25,000 I.U. of vitamin A, 1,000 mg of vitamin C in addition to a diet that supplied liberal amounts of wheat germ and Brewer's yeast. Although I had gained nearly 36 pounds (my usual weight is 110–115 pounds), by the time I delivered a healthy eight-pound girl, the stretch marks had actually improved, and after a few more months of intense treatment they nearly disappeared.

Vitamin E has been credited with preventing scar tissue from forming in individuals using large amounts of vitamin E externally and internally. My experience is that scars will not form if: (1) vitamin E is supplied generously and continuously inside and out, and (2) if the incision or injury is not in an area where stretching occurs easily (back of knee, elbow, etc.), thus preventing quick healing.

A PROVEN REMEDY FOR UGLY WARTS

I started my teenage years with an ugly, big wart on my right hand, and the customary handshake became utterly embarrassing. Over the years I tried everything from minor surgery over electrotherapy to silver nitrate application and the various herbal remedies, but after each successful removal the wart grew back. To this day I remember the hope each prospective cure initiated and the depression that followed after each failure.

Then one day an old acquaintance of Mother's noticed how I awkwardly tried to hide my hand, and because she insisted I showed her the disfiguring wart. Of course Mother told her about all the useless treatment programs I had tried and how discouraged I was. "My dear girl," the old lady said, "quit worrying. I know exactly what you should do." And she told me to apply chalk—simple white chalk—to the wart every night. Nothing else. I certainly thought that this was another old wives' tale, but I tried it nevertheless. What else was there to do? On the sixth night the wart fell off, and best of all, it never came back.

Several months ago my daughter noticed a good-sized wart on her right foot underneath the large toe. We applied chalk and a week later the wart had disappeared. Needless to say, it is gone for good.

HANDLING FUNGUS PROBLEMS WITH MONEY-SAVING REMEDIES

Fungus infections can develop under fingernails, around the genitals and anus, and on fingers and toes. An infection in the latter area is commonly referred to as athlete's foot.

Twenty-three-year-old Julie M. bitterly complained about a fungus problem that had developed around her vagina, causing much discomfort. She had tried antibiotics and numerous salves with no result, leaving her desperate. I recommended a combination of old and new remedies that I had tried the previous year to rid myself of an athlete's foot infection.

The treatment is simple. Take six or more acidophilus capsules, two to three high-potency vitamin B-complex tablets, one multivitamin supplement, one gram of vitamin C, and 400 I.U. of vitamin E daily. Soak once daily in a camomile/thyme sitz bath and drink one cup of thyme tea per day. To make the tea, add one teaspoon of thyme to one cup hot water, steep three to five minutes, and strain.

I also told her to apply plain yogurt to the affected area, and wear white panties only. Since vaginal infections are often aggravated by the use of colored toilet tissue, I insisted that she avoid all contact with colored paper or garments.

Julie followed the program and soon her problem improved and eventually disappeared.

INDIAN AND OTHER REMEDIES FOR HERPES INFECTIONS AND SKIN ERUPTIONS

Herpes infections are characterized by water blisters that appear as cold sores or fever blisters around the mouth and nose, the hands, abdomen, and the genitals. Because herpes flare-ups are sometimes linked to stress, following the stress treatment program (outlined in Chapter 6) may improve the condition and prevent outbreaks. The addition of 15 to 50 mg of zinc also helps healing.

The old Indian pokeweed treatment is raising interest among scientists. This wild plant grows in the northeastern and southeastern parts of the United States, has been investigated by a team of microbiologists at Southwest Texas State University in San Marcos, Texas, as a possible herpes virus inhibitor. The protein found in the plant, studies indicate, has proven effective as an antiviral agent that attacks a wide range of viruses, including herpes, influenza, and polio. Best of all, the advantage of pokeweed protein is that the concentration needed to inhibit virus multiplication is not toxic to cells. Though pokeweed protein is easily isolated via laboratory procedures, it is not yet commercially available.

Cooked and canned pokeweed leaves provide small amounts of pokeweed protein. It is interesting that the Indians and Appalachians have for years favored this vegetable, which resembles and tastes like spinach.

When blisters appear, a pokeweed poultice (see previous section on "Indian Remedy for Cancerous Ulcers") brings quick relief. A pokeweed infusion also alleviates this and other skin problems.

Pokeweed Infusion

Add 1 teaspoon dried young leaves to 1 pint boiling-hot water, simmer for 5 minutes and strain. Take 1 cup in mouthful doses throughout the day.

Applying raw potato slices or fresh garlic to lip sores also speeds up healing. When the sores have opened, zinc ointment helps clear the condition. While fresh garlic (cut bulb in half and rub onto affected area) applied to lip sores can be unpleasant, it works. I have tried it many times and the cold sores, which normally remain an unpleasant sight for one to two weeks, healed in one-half to one-third of that time.

REDUCING "OLD-AGE SPOTS"

Aloe vera gel, comfrey pulp, or European centaury juice, applied to the skin, have reportedly reduced discolorations called "old-age spots" or other skin pigmentations.

To make the comfrey pulp (*Symphytum officinalis*), add sufficient water to freshly grated or dried powdered rootstock to form a thick paste and apply this to skin. Remove paste after 15 minutes, cleanse area with lukewarm water, and rub diluted lemon juice onto affected area.

European centaury juice can be made by using the fresh herb only.

Cut one cup of the herb in small pieces, add to juicer containing one-half cup of water. Juice the herb and use as skin lotion.

Taken internally, vitamin A and E also help improve the condition.

PREVENTING AND TREATING WRINKLES

Beaten egg whites make an excellent facial mask that tightens and tones the skin. Another common household item and favorite European beauty aid is homemade mayonnaise. It is a marvelous skin softener, and like a warm oil facial, it regenerates the skin by supplying natural oils and needed nutrients.

Egg White Facial Mask

Beat egg whites and apply to freshly cleansed skin. Leave on for 15 to 20 minutes and wash off with lukewarm water and follow with a cold rinse.

Mayonnaise Facial

To make a mayonnaise facial, add one egg, one teaspoon honey, and one-half to one teaspoon of apple cider vinegar to blender and mix for one minute at medium speed. Continue blending and slowly add sunflower or olive oil until mixture is thickened.

Spread a thin layer over clean face and leave on for 15 to 20 minutes. Remove with lukewarm water by using facial tissue and sprinkle with liberal amounts of witch hazel decoction (see "Steaming Away Ugly Boils"). Rejuvenates dry skin.

My Favorite Wheat Germ Oil Facial

Use camomile vapor bath (see section on "Steaming Away Ugly Boils") to open pores and then cleanse skin with witch hazel decoction. Apply lukewarm wheat germ oil to face and throat, cover with warm, moist towel and leave on for 15 minutes while resting. (Reheat towel if necessary.) Remove oil with warm, wet washcloth and sprinkle with generous amounts of witch hazel decoction. Rejuvenates and smooths skin.

Biochemical research suggests that large doses of vitamin E can prevent premature aging of the skin. Lester Packer and James Smith from the University of California at Berkeley, and the Veterans Administration Hospital demonstrated that vitamin E intake doubled healthy cell production. What is even more fascinating is that these cells did behave like much younger cells, and when subjected to ultraviolet light and high oxygen toxicity, vitamin E actually protected these cells, which indicates that vitamin E plays an important role in the prevention of premature aging.

AIDING SUNBURN

Sunburn, also called dermatitis solaris, can be dangerous and extremely painful, resulting in blistering and even nausea and fainting. On top of it, sunburn can lead to spotting, aging, wrinkling, and worst of all, skin cancer.

Since the sun's ultraviolet rays cause all of these problems, the best prevention is to limit sun exposure, or intercept UV (ultraviolet) light between the sun and your skin. The B vitamin PABA (para-aminobenzoic acid) can do just that. Medical studies indicate that this vitamin is useful in the prevention and treatment of sunburns. Studies indicate that individuals who were especially prone to sunburns tolerated 50 to 100 times more exposure when taking 1,000 mg of PABA, and others who suffered from sunburn found great relief by applying lotions containing PABA.

After moving to Colorado, my husband sunburned quickly. I mixed about one-half to one teaspoon of PABA with water, which I then applied carefully (!) to sensitive and burned areas. It brought great relief. After taking zinc and PABA, internally and externally, my husband soon tolerated the sun better and tanned without burning.

Oral zinc therapy, DeWayne Ashmed, Ph.D. reports, greatly improves recovery from sunburns and other more serious burns. At the International Symposium on Zinc Metabolism, Dr. Luane Larson documented that zinc is essential to patients suffering from burns and if given in adequate amounts speeds up recovery.

Applying a paste of baking soda and cornstarch to sunburned areas also brings relief, as does aloe vera juice.

My uncle, Dr. Felix Hach, a medical doctor in Ankeny, Iowa, and a true sun lover, prevents the aches and pains of sunburns by taking a hot shower after extensive sunbathing. This desensitizes the skin, thus preventing pain. We tried it. It works.

EASY WAYS TO CORRECT EXCESSIVE SWEATING AND BODY ODORS

German studies point out that sage leaves (*Salvia officinalis*) have a calming effect on the sweat glands and effectively reduce excessive perspiration, whether it occurs in the underarm areas, the hands, feet, or the entire body. Sage leaves also strengthen the nervous system, and have been found useful in controlling fatigue due to puberty or menopause. German doctors often recommend sage to accelerate surgical recovery.

Since sage reduces sweat gland activity, nursing mothers are advised to stay away from this herb. For those who are weaning a child, sage tea or juice will actually stop the flow of milk.

Sage Leaf Tea

Add one teaspoon fresh or dried sage leaves to one cup hot water and steep for 10 to 30 minutes. Strain and drink one cup per day in small doses.

Sage Leaf Juice

This old-country remedy quickly controls excess perspiration. Collect fresh leaves before flowering time and add one handful of the herb to blender containing one-half to one cup of tomato juice. Blend until smooth and drink one cup per day.

The daily intake of a high-potency vitamin B complex not only relieves perspiration, but drastically reduces odors . I can testify to that. For years, stress caused me to perspire heavily under the armpits. No matter how often I bathed and showered, an odor developed as soon as I was under tension, and there was no antiperspirant that successfully concealed my problem, although baking soda mixed with baby powder helped somewhat. After I began to take one to two tablets of a high-potency B complex vitamin daily, the problem disappeared completely (to my great relief).

YOUR NAILS REVEAL YOUR STATE OF HEALTH

Biochemical studies indicate that rhythmic patterns of white spots or bands on the fingernails reflect low zinc levels and often correspond with menstrual cycles in women, which, due to the change in hormone levels, often cause a drop in serum zinc and a rise in serum copper. Similar mineral imbalances and corresponding nail problems can also be observed in individuals with a high estrogen intake.

Women using birth control pills often have brittle nails, and the same phenomenon occurs in men subjected to estrogen therapy. As soon as the diet contains adequate supplies of protein, zinc, and sulfur, nail growth becomes normal.

Serious colds, viral infections, inadequate diets, fasting, or other severe stresses can also result in zinc and other nutritional deficiencies which cause nail abnormalities. When 15 mg or more of zinc are given to individuals with nail abnormalities, nail growth returns to normal. Since an adult's nail growth is between 0.104 and 0.108 mm per day, it takes approximately five to six months before nails are completely replaced. By the same token, today's zinc deficiency or injury becomes noticeable about four weeks later as a white spot, furrow, or other nail problem.

Opaque nails marked by wavy patterns are often found in hypertensive individuals and others suffering from mineral imbalances. When zinc and vitamin B-6 are introduced, the color of the nails returns to a healthy pink again.

Since nails are made of protein, fingernails that are extremely thin, fail to grow, or split or break easily, generally indicate a protein deficiency or inadequate vitamin A intake, or both. Sulfur, which is also extremely important to normal nail and hair growth, is mostly supplied by food protein, namely eggs, meat, and garlic.

European health spas such as Baden near Vienna, Bad Goisern southeast of Salzburg, and others employ sulfur therapy to correct skin, nail, and hair problems, but if you cannot afford a four-week stay at one of these marvelous spas, take zinc sulfate, garlic, and a vitamin B-complex containing vitamin B-6. Within a few months' time you will be blessed with healthy nails, hair, and skin.

Brittle or thin nails recover quicker when soaked in lukewarm wheat germ oil. Warm the oil slightly and soak nails for five to ten minutes each day. Wipe off excess oil and massage nails from top down.

The case of young Eric is most interesting and underlines biochemical research that indicates that adolescent males are often extremely deficient in zinc and other nutrients. Zinc deficiencies are often the cause of stunted growth in males.

Eric was bothered by ugly, ingrown toenails. He decided to try the external and internal treatment as outlined above. Not only did his nail growth return to normal; the boy who used to be considerably smaller than average noticed a spurt in growth rate, for which he was extremely grateful.

GRANDMA'S REMEDY FOR BRITTLE EYELASHES

Everybody adores long, shiny eyelashes and the cosmetic industry is working hard to promote mascara that adds length and color to conscientious, beauty-seeking consumers. Unfortunately, what you see on TV is not necessarily what you get. In other words, adding mascara to short, brittle eyelashes may provide you (and others) with a few hours of illusion, but despite commercial promises, cannot eliminate the problem.

Yet there is no need to despair. Do what many of my friends and I did. Try Grandma's old-fashioned treatment that is simple, inexpensive, and works like a charm. Each night, apply castor oil to clean eyelashes and you will soon enjoy long, silky eyelashes.

CUSTOMARY EUROPEAN TREATMENTS FOR HEALTHIER HAIR

Everybody likes healthy hair—lots of it—and while genetics largely determine hair color and thickness, proper health and hair care helps you to enjoy your natural crown for much longer. Thinning hair, dry skin, and brittle nails are often signs of an underactive thyroid, or these symptoms may be signs of other hormonal imbalances or nutritional deficiencies.

Hair is made of protein and minerals, therefore a diet adequate in these and other needed nutrients is necessary for proper hair growth. Animal studies suggest that a lack of magnesium and the B vitamins results in hair loss. Premature graying has reportedly been linked to a number of nutritional deficiencies, including the lack of PABA (para-aminobenzoic acid), pantothenic acid, copper and folic acid. In some cases, the correction of specific nutritional imbalances has restored to the patients their original hair color.

Since high-fashion hair products occasionally turn out to be disastrous to the health of your hair, natural hair treatments are more in vogue than ever, and if you are dissatisfied with the shade of your hair, old-time herbal rinses provide you with a safe and natural alternative.

For Blondes and Redheads

A lemon hair rinse adds sunshine to hair. Use the strained juice of two to three lemons, dilute with one cup of warm water, and apply to hair. If you leave the rinse on and sit in the sunshine for 10 to 20 minutes, your hair will turn lighter. Rinse with plenty of warm water.

Roman camomile (*Anthemis nobilis*) also makes a wonderful rinse that highlights and somewhat lightens the hair. It's my favorite. Add one cup of this herb to one pint of hot water, steep for 10 minutes, and strain. Use as final rinse.

Linden or lime flowers (*Tilia officinalis*) make a mildly bleaching, antiseptic rinse that stimulates circulation and hair growth. Use in the same way as the Roman camomile rinse.

Beauty stores now carry natural henna products again. Henna rinses, which have been used for millenia to produce exotic shades of red, are available to those desiring special effects.

For Brunettes

Sage (*Salvia officinalis*) darkens the hair. Add one-third of a cup of sage leaves to one quart water. Steep two hours and strain. Pour into bowl and soak hair. Leave on for one-half hour and rinse with plenty of warm water.

For Thinning Hair

Mix one ounce of rosemary with one ounce of linden flowers. Prepare like the Roman camomile rinse, apply to hair, and massage into scalp.

For Dry and Thinning Hair

Massage castor oil into scalp. Use steaming hot towel, wrap around head, and leave on for one-half hour. Thoroughly shampoo hair and rinse with rosemary/linden decoction.

For Dandruff

Mix 1 oz. fennel seeds (*Foeniculum vulgare*)
1 oz. Roman camomile (*Anthemis nobilis*)
1 oz. rosemary (*Rosmarinus officinalis*)
1 oz. oak bark (*Quercus alba*)
1 oz. walnut leaves (*Juglans regia*)
1 oz. willow bark (*Salix alba*)

Add five tablespoons of herbal mixture to one quart cold water, bring to boil, and simmer for 10 minutes. Strain and drink two to three cups per day. Use the rest as an herbal rinse.

****

References:

Airola, Paavo O., N.D., Ph.D. *How to Keep Slim, Healthy and Young With Juice Fasting.* Health Plus Publ., 1971.

Blaurock-Busch, Eleonore. "Natural Treatment for Acne." *Bestways.* Dec. 1980, pp. 88–89.

————. "Hot Packs: Ancient Natural Therapy." *Bestways.* Jan. 1981, pp. 102–104.

Furlenmeier, M., M.D. *Wunderwelt der Heilpflanzen.* Zurich: Schwitter Holding, 1978.

Goerz, Heinz, W. *Gesundheit durch Heilkraüter.* Wiesbaden: Moeller Verl., 1974.

Krochmal, Arnold and Connie. *A Guide to Medicinal Plants.* Quadrangle/York Times Book Co., 1973.

Kugler, Hans J., Ph.D. *Dr. Kugler's Seven Keys to a Longer Life.* Stein & Day, 1978.

Kunz-Bircher, Ruth. *The Bircher-Benner Health Guide.* Santa Barbara, Cal.: Woodbridge Press, 1980.

Lindt, Inge. *Naturheilkunde.* Koeln: Buch und Zeit Verlag, 1977.

Lust, John B., N.D., D.B.M. *The Herb Book.* Bantam Book, 1974

Pfeiffer, Carl C., M.D., Ph.D. *Mental and Elemental Nutrients.* Keats, 1975.

Schauenberg, P.; Paris, F. *BLV Bestimmungsbuch, Heilpflanzen.* 3rd ed., Munich: BLV, 1978.

Stage, Wolfgang, M.D. *Das Kneipp Taschenbuch.* Ullstein, 1968.

8

Taking Care of Your Teeth with Old-Fashioned, Easy-to-Make Dental Products

HEALTHY TEETH FOR A LIFETIME

Despite regular checkups and fluoridation, 35 percent of the American people are toothless by 60 years of age. The villain is not so much dental decay, but periodontal disease, which, unfortunately, often proceeds unrecognized until damage is severe. Consequently, treatment of advanced periodontal disease is extensive, painful, and expensive, costing an average of $1,500 or more.

How do you recognize periodontal disease? In its early stages, this dental problem is referred to as gingivitis. Gums or soft tissues are inflammed, swollen, and bleed easily, though little or no pain is present. Bad breath may develop and pus or discharge may be noticeable between gums and teeth. Gum shrinkage or pockets between teeth and gums can cause loosening of teeth, and changes in the fit of bridgework or partials may be an indication of early dental disease. If these early symptoms are ignored, plaque bacteria resume their devastating process, causing greater shrinkage of gum tissue and the formation of additional plaque deposits. Over the years, gum tissues deteriorate, ultimately resulting in the loosening and eventual loss of healthy teeth.

According to Dr. Robert O. Nara, new research in odontosism, the term applied to initial dental disease, indicates that certain germs are at the base of all dental diseases, creating bad breath and the unpleasant taste and "furry" feel of the tooth surface. New tests such as the saliva and Navy Plaque Index Test, Dr. Nara says, help evaluate and control periodontal disease, helping patients understand the severity of the problem. Ask your dentist about these tests or write to: Oramedicas International Laboratory, Canton, Ohio, for more information.

Simple preventive measures such as good dental hygiene and proper eating habits certainly help protect your healthy set of teeth. Avoiding sweets, brushing after meals and using dental floss are excellent defenses against dental disease. Add to this program, old-fashioned, natural dental products that effectively attack villainous bacteria, and your self-defense program is better than ever. But best of all, you can make many of these dental remedies that used to be prepared in German druggists' laboratories right in the privacy of your own kitchen—for just a few pennies a product. Experiment. It's fun. If you wonder about where to get the required ingredients, inquire at your local drugstore, grocery, and health foods store and you'll soon be ready to prepare the dental products that suit your individual needs.

MY FATHER'S OLD-TIME DENTAL PRODUCTS

I treasure my father's old books. I call them survival manuals, for they have taught me to make almost anything. Are you interested in making your own tooth fillings? Not really? How about your own toothpaste or toothache remedy? Father's books can tell you how. They are full of old-time recipes that used to be prepared in druggists' laboratories long before my apprentice years, and though modern products eventually replaced natural ingredients with artificial ones, the basic recipes have hardly changed. At a time where synthetics conquer our daily lives and where going back to nature becomes more and more necessary to good health, using original, natural products only makes sense.

TRADITIONAL RECIPES FOR HOMEMADE TOOTHPASTE

Granted, you have to be dedicated to natural living to make your own toothpaste, especially since natural products are now found in many American health food stores, but if you are an experimenter, try my father's recipe for homemade toothpaste. It came in handy during wartime when everything was scarce and, in case you haven't noticed, this book is a late thank you to my innovative and handy parents whose resources protected us from starvation, the all-too-common destiny of war victims.

Certainly, the majority of the people living during WWII were too hungry to be concerned about dental hygiene and understandably showed more interest in filling their stomachs than in buying or trading valuables for toothpaste. But as in any war, there were also those who had plenty of food. Most farmers, for instance, did not suffer. Most had plenty and they drove a hard bargain for an egg, a couple of potatoes, a handful of grain, or a cup of milk and it was not unusual for people to exchange a complete set of silverware or elegant linen for one head of cabbage. To this day many Germans, Mother included, are bitter towards greedy farmers who rather saw food rot than share it with the needy. Of course, when those farmers required help for their livestock, needed soap or even toothpaste, a druggists's know-how came in handy. As a result, I, unlike other war children, did not suffer and Mother's knowledge (Father was an officer in the army and later a prisoner of war in Russia) helped us and others survive. For when we had food, we shared. Mother distributed food and clothing among the poor and she never cared who they were or what their political conviction, race, or religion was. It was simple. The hungry were fed and the cold were clothed, and to this day there are many who are truly grateful. Even farmers admire her gutsy survival instinct, her knowledge, and dedication.

Following are some old-fashioned basic recipes for toothpastes, the true forerunners of today's glamorous products.

Mint-Flavored Toothpaste

200 grams calcium carbonate
100 grams brown or green soft soap (not the modern kind now sold
   in fancy bottles that contains all sorts of chemical ingredients.
   The soft soap needed here as a foaming agent for toothpastes is
   made from animal fats or vegetable oils and potash lye only)
50 grams magnesium carbonate
5 milliliters menthol
Mix ingredients and slowly add 100 to 150 milliliters of glycerin until
paste is formed. Fill container with toothpaste.

Herbal Toothpaste

5 oz. calcium carbonate
2 ½ oz. soft soap
1 oz. magnesium carbonate
1 oz. myrrh tincture
1 oz. olive oil
10–20 drops peppermint oil
⅓ oz. glycerin
3 drops thymol
½ oz. alcohol (75%)
Mix all ingredients into smooth paste and fill in container.

Soap-Free Toothpaste

8 oz. diatomaceous earth (diatomite)
3 oz. alum
3 oz. glycerin
1½ oz. myrrh powder

Mix ingredients into smooth paste and flavor with peppermint, wintergreen, anise, fennel, clove or any other herbal oil or tincture you prefer.

EUROPEAN TOOTH POWDERS FOR SPARKLING TEETH

Long before toothpaste became popular, tooth powders were commonly used to brighten teeth and to freshen the breath. Their advantage? They are mildly abrasive without damaging the teeth's enamel, and this superior cleansing action is particularly useful to stained teeth as seen in smokers or heavy coffee drinkers. In addition, tooth powders can be quickly prepared by anyone anywhere. Try these fabulous old-time products, and you too may say goodbye to commercial toothpaste.

Old-Fashioned Tooth Powder

Mix and keep in closed container:
200 grams calcium carbonate
2 drops peppermint oil (more if desired)
1 drop vanillin

or

200 grams calcium carbonate
15 grams magnesium carbonate
10 drops thymol
2 drops peppermint oil

Herbal Tooth Powder

2 cups calcium carbonate or baking soda
1 oz. sweet flag rootstock, powdered
1 oz. peppermint leaves, powdered, or 5 drops peppermint oil, or
    10–15 drops mint extract
⅓ oz. sage leaves, powdered
⅓ oz. flag lily rootstock, powdered
5 drops menthol (can be replaced with 20 drops or more of mint
    extract)

Northern European Tooth Powder for Whiter Teeth

1 cup baking soda
1–2 tablespoons sea salt
2–5 drops peppermint oil, anise oil, clove oil, or 10 drops wintergreen or cinnamon extract. (The addition of 1 teaspoon cinnamon powder improves taste and color.)
or

> 1 cup baking soda
> 2 tablespoons powdered flag lily rootstock and/or 5 drops menthol,
> peppermint oil or vanillin (use any flavor you like).
> Mix ingredients and keep in closed container.

Experiment with different flavors (vanillin, mint, etc.) to create your very own naturally flavored tooth powder. Set your imagination free and let your taste buds be the final judge. Of course, you could use food coloring to add more of a special touch to the powder, but if you are concerned about artificial colorings as I am, you will focus on taste rather than looks. What about decorating the powder with fresh mint leaves?

If you need a special gift for a beauty- and health-conscious friend, learn from the cosmetic industry. Find an elegant container for your product, and violà, you have an innovative and attractive present. Have you considered going into business? The market is wide open for natural products.

EASY-TO-MAKE OLD-COUNTRY MOUTHWASHES AND GARGLES

Do you need a tasty and effective mouthwash? Well, who doesn't? Judging by the commercial success of gargles and mouthwashes such products are always appreciated.

Gargles and mouthwashes are made easily. There are two basic formulas and either one is simple to follow.

Formula 1: Use 2 to 4 oz. of any of the herbs listed below, soak in 1 cup ethyl alcohol (75% proof) for a week, strain, and dilute with 2 cups distilled water.

Formula 2: Add herbal extracts, tinctures, or oils to 1 cup ethyl alcohol (75% proof), dilute with 1–2 cups of distilled water and shake well.

Herbs for Mouthwashes

• Aaron's rod (*Sempervivum tectorum*)—astringent; good for inflammations

• Agrimony (*Agrimonia eupatoria*)—astringent; good for receding gums, bleeding gums; promotes healing; use after tooth extraction

• Almond extract (*Prunus amydalus*)—aromatic flavoring; soothes pain

• Althea or marshmallow root (*Althaea officinalis*)—good for inflamed and irritated tissues

• Anise seeds (*Pimpinella anisum*)—aromatic flavoring; reduces pain

- Camomile (*Matricaria chamomilla*)—reduces pain and inflammation, promotes healing; excellent after tooth extraction or oral surgery
- Cankerroot (*Coptis trifolia*)—good for inflammations, sores, ulcers
- Cardamom (*Elettaria cardamomum*)—flavoring
- Cinnamon (*Cinnamomum cassia* or *C. zeylanicum*)—flavoring
- Cloves (*Caryophyllus aromaticus* or *Syzygium aromaticum*)—reduces pain; kills germs; promotes healing
- Comfrey (*Symphytum officinale*)—astringent; relieves pain; good for sore throats, inflammations, hoarseness and bleeding gums
- Eucalyptus (*Eucalyptus globulus*)—antiseptic
- European angelica root (*Angelica archangelica*)—relieves pain, promotes healing
- Fenugreek (*Trigonella foenum-graecum*)—for inflammations, sore throats, tumors, sores, fistulas
- Goldenseal (*Hydrastis canadensis*)—antiseptic; astringent; good for infections and fungus problems such as thrush
- Lady's mantle (*Alchemilla vulgaris*)—astringent; tonic; good for inflammations; stops bleeding; use after tooth extraction
- Lemon (*Citrus limon*)—adds fresh taste; good for bleeding gums
- Lemon balm (*Melissa officinalis*)—freshens breath; helps toothaches
- Marigold (*Calendula officinalis*)—helps gum inflammations
- Menthol (obtained from mint oil)—strong antiseptic; flavoring known for its cooling taste; breath freshener; promotes healing
- Mullein (*Verbascum thapsiforme*)—relieves pain and inflammation
- Myrrh (*Commiphora myrrha*)—antiseptic; astringent; good for gum inflammations and all dental problems
- Peppermint (*Mentha piperita*)—flavoring; antiseptic; promotes healing of sores and ulcers; breath freshener
- Plantain (*Plantago lanceolato*)—helps inflammations, bleeding gums, toothaches
- Rose oil or extract (*Rosa canina*)—flavoring; astringent; good for mouth sores and thrush
- Sage (*Salvia officinalis*)—strong astringent; reduces saliva production; good for all gum problems
- Sandalwood (*Santalum album*)—astringent; disinfectant; good for all inflammations and infections
- Shave grass (*Equisetum arvense*)—stops bleeding; good after dental surgery; improves healing; prevents scar tissue formation
- Sweet flag root (*Acorus calamus*)—mildly sedating; reduces pain and gum problems

• Tarragon (*Artemisia dracunculus*)—flavoring
• Thyme (*Thymus vulgaris*)—antiseptic; flavoring; good for infections
• Thymol (obtained from thyme oil)—strong and effective antiseptic
• Vanillin extract (*Vanilla aromatica*)—flavoring
• Wild geranium (*Geranium maculatum*)—astringent; good for receding and bleeding gums
• White oak bark (*Quercus alba*)—astringent, tonic; strengthens gum tissue
• Wintergreen (*Gaultheria procumbens*)—analgesic; astringent; strengthens gum tissue; reduces pain and inflammations

Antiseptic Gargles and Mouthwashes

Eucalyptus Mouthwash and Gargle

Combine and shake:
1 cup alcohol (75% proof)
½ cup distilled water
1 tablespoon eucalyptus oil
1 teaspoon peppermint oil

Mint-Flavored Mouthwash and Gargle

1 cup alcohol (75% proof)
1 cup distilled water
1 teaspoon wintergreen oil
1 teaspoon peppermint oil

or

Strong Antiseptic (use sparingly)

1 cup alcohol (75% proof)
½ to 1 cup distilled water
1 teaspoon thymol
1 teaspoon menthol

Popular Oriental Mouthwash
(good breath freshener)

2 cups distilled water
½ cup alcohol (75% proof)
2 drops rose oil
2 drops peppermint oil
2 drops anise oil
1–3 drops vanillin extract

Additional flavors to be used are: anise, clove, almond, and lemon oil or extract. The addition of thymol and menthol, both of which are strong antiseptics, makes good germ-killing mouthwashes and mouth fresheners.

Listerine Substitute

2 cups distilled water
1 cup alcohol (75% proof)
1 tablespoon boric acid
5 drops eucalyptus oil
5 drops wintergreen oil
5 drops menthol
5 drops thymol

Combine ingredients and shake well.

Nonalcoholic Antiseptic Mouthwashes

2 oz. eucalyptus leaves
2 oz. lemon balm
2 oz. peppermint leaves
2 oz. plantain
2 oz. sage leaves
2 oz. thyme

or

2 oz. aniseed
2 oz. cardamom
2 oz. cloves
2 oz. sage leaves
2 oz. sandalwood
2 oz. sweet flag root

Boil 3 tablespoons of herbal mixture in 1 pint water for 10 minutes. Steep for an additional 10 minutes and strain. Best used warm.

Grandma's Simple Mouthwash for Inflammations, Sores and Ulcers

1 oz. cankerroot
1 oz. cloves
1 oz. German camomile
1 oz. peppermint leaves
1 oz. white oak bark
1 oz. wild geranium
1 oz. wintergreen

Prepare like nonalcoholic antiseptic mouthwashes, add 1 teaspoon table salt to 1 cup mouthwash and gargle three to four times daily.

OLD-WORLD REMEDIES FOR TOOTHACHES

It's three a.m. and you are suddenly hit by a devastating toothache. You call the dentist, yet you can't get past the answering service which assures you that the doctor will call you first thing in the morning. Don't get upset. There is really no need to wish the plague on the poor doctor's family, or pump painkillers into your stomach. Try an old druggist's remedy instead. It will soothe your aches and get you back to sleep in a hurry.

Rinse your mouth with an antiseptic mouthwash. Soak a piece of cotton with clove oil or myrrh tincture and apply to the hurting tooth. This quickly reduces pain.

German dentists also recommend aspirin for localized aches, but instead of swallowing the pill, crush it and smear the powder in or around the hurting tooth. This clever treatment alleviates aches without upsetting the stomach. If you are allergic to aspirin, which many people are, don't try this remedy. Even though you avoid swallowing the drug, minute amounts will be ingested into your system and possibly trigger an allergic reaction.

Swiss country folks use fresh horseradish poultices to alleviate the pain of major toothaches, headaches, and neuralgias. According to Dr. Furlenmaier, this old-country remedy works like a charm. Grate fresh horseradish root and spread on a hot cloth. Apply to sensitive area and wrap towel around to retain moisture. Remove after 30 minutes.

My favorite remedy for toothaches and inflammations, which is especially suitable for children and old people, is the camomile compress. Prepare a hot camomile infusion to soak a clean cloth or wash towel, wring out excess moisture, and apply to affected areas as hot as can be borne comfortably by the patient. Leave on until cold and repeat until relieved.

EUROPEAN TEETHING AID FOR INFANTS

Dried flag lily rootstock (*Iris germanica*) is probably one of the oldest teething aids, having been used by European country folks for centuries. It's a marvelous and tasty remedy and mothers and infants still prefer it to plastic rings and other such teething aids. Just test your youngster. Let him chew on a dried flag lily rootstock for awhile. Then replace it with a plastic ring. If your child is like mine, you'll hear some protesting.

For ages, cut, peeled, and dried lily rootstock, which is typical for its aromatic flavor, has been sold in German drugstores. String one or more together and your child will have much fun playing with and chewing on Mother Nature's tasty teething aid.

Rubbing the gums with orange mullein oil (*Verbascum phlomoides* or *V. thapsiforme*) or marigold juice (*Calendula officinalis*), freshly made from flower heads, also brings relief.

WHAT TO DO ABOUT THRUSH

This discomforting oral disease, caused by a fungus, is recognizable by white patches which commonly appear in the mouths of infants. Traditionally, German folk healers recommend that older children frequently gargle with a camomile/sage/shave grass decoction. To make this remedy, mix together one ounce of each herb. Add one tablespoon of this herbal mixture to one cup boiling-hot water and steep for five to ten minutes. Strain and gargle repeatedly.

Rose honey with borax is another old-fashioned German remedy that is commonly used to treat thrush and other gum problems in small infants. It has been around as long as my grandmother could remember and continues to be marketed in drugstores throughout the country. Today's young mothers still use it in the same fashion their mothers and grandmothers did centuries ago.

While it is simplest to use commercially marketed products, a somewhat modified remedy can be prepared in the kitchen.

> Add 1 oz. crushed rose petal leaves to 5 oz. diluted alcohol. Close container and store for 24 hours at room temperature. Shake occasionally. Filter and pour liquid into a pot holding 9 oz. honey. Boil down to 9 or 10 oz. until all the alcohol has evaporated. Dissolve 1 oz. boric acid in sufficient warm water and stir into rose honey. Let mixture cool down and apply to affected area with a small brush.

Country folks also used a decoction of white oak bark, myrrh, and goldenseal (containing boric acid) to swab affected areas. This remedy, which enjoyed great popularity, continues to be used by many with good results.

Herbal Decoction for Thrush

2 oz. oak bark
2 oz. myrrh
1 oz. goldenseal

Use: Add 2 tablespoons herbal mixture to 1 pint cold water and bring to boil. Simmer for 10 minutes, strain, add 1 teaspoon boric acid to decoction and let stand for 30 minutes. Apply to affected area.

Supplementing the diet with vitamins A, B and C, and the mineral zinc also helps to alleviate thrush and other dental diseases.

ANCIENT WAYS TO CONTROL GUM PROBLEMS

Myrrh (*Commiphora myrrha*) is one of the oldest herbal remedies which, as has been pointed out in the Bible, has long been treasured as if it were gold. In Europe, myrrh tincture is considered a most effective herbal remedy for dental problems, including sore and inflamed gums, receding and bleeding gums, loose teeth, even bad breath. Rub a few drops of myrrh tincture on troubled gums each day and you will soon notice an improvement in dental health.

A myrrh infusion makes an excellent and effective antiseptic and astringent mouthwash that is useful for gum and throat infections. Steep one teaspoon of myrrh in one pint of boiling-hot water for 10 minutes, strain and add one teaspoon of boric acid. Let stand for 20 to 30 minutes and gargle.

Bleeding gums respond well to an old German herbal mouthwash consisting of equal parts of:

> agrimony
> lady's mantle
> oak bark
> sage
> Use: Add 2 teaspoons of the herbal mixture to 1 pint cold water and soak for 1 hour. Bring to quick boil, remove from heat, and steep for 10 minutes. Strain and gargle.

Rubbing the gums with powdered oak bark or fresh oak leaf juice also brings quick improvement and soon firms gums and teeth. Smokers who often are afflicted with periodontal disease that is caused by nutritional deficiencies benefit from the above treatment, especially when used in conjunction with vitamin C therapy. According to Dr. Donsbach of Donsbach University, Huntington Beach, California, all smokers, whether they are afflicted with gum problems or not, should supplement their diets with vitamin C.

OLD HERBAL REMEDIES FOR MOUTH ULCERS
AND CANKER SORES

Ulcers, German folk healers and phytotherapists insist, are best treated with an old-fashioned mouthwash that is made of equal parts of:

Aaron's rod
althea root
fenugreek
sage

Use: Add 1 teaspoon herbal mixture to 1 cup cold water and let soak for 1 to 2 hours. Bring to quick boil, add 1 teaspoon camomile flowers and immediately remove from heat. Strain after 5 minutes and use warm or cold, but gargle repeatedly.

In addition, swabbing sores and ulcers with dilute myrrh tincture speeds up the healing process.

FRESHEN YOUR BREATH NATURALLY

Bad breath, like acne, won't kill you but it sure can ruin your love life, and that is a shame because generally, this problem is easily corrected. Chewing dill seeds helps halitosis (another term for bad breath), and chlorophyll/thymol tablets sold in health food stores quickly freshen the worst breath. Chew one or two tablets after you eat strong foods or (heaven forbid) drink or smoke, and your mouth will feel as clean as a spring breeze.

The following old-time herbal breath freshener tea improves digestive problems which often are the underlying cause of halitosis. In addition to taking the above mentioned chlorophyll/thymol tablets and chewing dill seeds, drink two to three cups of this tea throughout the day and soon you won't hear any complaints about your breath.

Herbal Breath Freshener Tea

1 oz. anise
1 oz. camomile
1 oz. peppermint leaves
1 oz. lemon balm
½ oz. European angelica root
½ oz. echinacea
½ oz. cloves
½ oz. parsley

Add 1 teaspoon of herbal mixture to 1 cup cold water and soak for 1 hour. Bring to boil, remove from heat, and strain after 5 minutes.

Take Susie C., who suffered from a severe case of halitosis that was relieved only temporarily by strong mouthwashes advertised on TV. After years of discomfort, she started this old-time herbal program and within a week her problem disappeared. Talk about happiness!

******

References:

Buchheister-Ottersbach. *Vorschriftenbuch fuer Drogisten.* Julius Springer Verlag, 1914.

Cheraskin, E., M.D., D.M.D.; Ringsdorf, W.M., Jr., D.M.D.; Clark, J.W., D.D.S. *Diet and Disease.* Keats, 1968.

Freise, Ed, Ph.D.; Von Morgenstern, F., Ph.D. *Der Drogist, Band I & II.* Heinrich Killinger Verlag.

Furlenmaier, M., M.D. *Wunderwelt der Heilpflanzen.* Zurich: Schwitter Holding, 1978.

Goerz, Heinz. *Gesundheit durch Heilkraeuter.* Wilhelm Moeller Verlag, 1974.

Heinerman, John. *Science of Herbal Medicine.* By-World, 1979.

Lindt, Inge. *Naturheilkunde, Heilkraeuter und ihre Anwendung, Krankheiten und ihre Behandlung.* Buch und Zeit Verlag, 1977.

Lust, John B., N.D., D.B.M. *The Herb Book.* Bantam Books, 1974.

Nara, Robert O., D.D.S.; Mariner, Steven S. "Doctor, Please Don't Hurt Me." *Today's Chiropractic.* August 1981, pp. 19, 20.

Patterson, Donald Ray. "Ways You Can Prevent Periodontal Disease." *Bestways.* Sept. 1979, pp. 75–79.

Rettenmaier, Rudolf; Rissmann, Adolf, Ph.D. *Lehrbuch fuer Drogisten, Band I.* Rudolf Mueller Verlag, 1962.

Rettenmaier; Rissmann; Ziegler, Ph.D.s. *Botanik-Drogenkunde.* Rudolf Mueller Verlag, 1975.

Schauenberg, P.; Paris, F.; *BLV Bestimmungsbuch.* BLV Verlag, 1978.

Ziegler-Lander. *Drogistenpraxis.* Luitpold Lang Verlag, 1960.

9

Overcoming Earaches, Eye and Nose Problems as in Ancient Days

HOW I EASED MY DAUGHTER'S EARACHE

During her preschool years, our daughter, like many of her peers, was frequently troubled with earaches simply because she disliked wearing a hat during cold Colorado winter days.

In all instances camomile poultices eased the pain and quickly solved the problem. Only once was the pain so severe that I felt desperate. To make matters worse, after examining our daughter's ears, my husband suspected an ear infection plus a ruptured ear drum. Consequently, I took my daughter to a specialist who confirmed the diagnosis. After an extensive examination her ears were carefully cleaned of deposits, ear drops were inserted, and we were given a prescription for a 10-day oral antibiotic treatment. Although I am very fond of this doctor, the idea of treating a minor ear infection with antibiotics, which can do little to heal the rupture, did not appeal to me. But since I've been brought up not to argue with men (including doctors) I took the prescription anyhow, went straight home and applied my favorite camomile packs (see Chapter 8) which I frequently alternated with potato poultices—my mother-in-law's favorite old-time remedy.

Yvette's individual nutritional program included two garlic oil capsules to be taken four times daily for the first three days. For the following three days this dose was reduced to a total of six capsules and after that was further reduced to four capsules per day. In addition, I mixed one-third to one-half of a tablespoon of ascorbic acid with one glass of grape juice and gave this to her three to five times per day. This equalled a daily vitamin C intake of 3 to 7.5 grams per day. After signs of diarrhea appeared, vitamin C was removed from her diet and Yvette was given burned toast to stop the symptoms. Part of this temporary supplemental program were 50,000 International Units of vitamin A for the first three days and 20,000 I.U. thereafter. She also took a high-potency B-complex and a calcium supplement twice daily.

Within two days there was no more pain and discomfort. When we went for the follow-up visit with the ear specialist he was pleased and amazed at the progress she had made. There were no more signs of an infection and the ear drum had healed.

Grandma's Potato Poultice for Ear Infections

Boil several whole potatoes in plain water. Fold into clean cloths and shape into flat pack. Apply hot to affected ear, but let patient decide what feels comfortable. Remove when cold and reheat for additional applications. Can be reused two to three times.

FIGHTING INFECTIONS WITH AN OLD-FASHIONED ANTIBIOTIC

Garlic is one of the most effective natural antibiotics and, in the opinion of European botanists and phytotherapists, has a clear advantage over penicillin and other such antibiotics because instead of killing all bacteria, good and bad, garlic actually provides a better environment for the "good" bacteria, which help fight the "bad" guys. To demonstrate the effectiveness of garlic, repeat a simple experiment: place crushed garlic along with some bacterial culture or fungus under a glass dish, and watch the microorganism perish within a few minutes.

Garlic has long been recognized as a valuable antiseptic and has been used by people throughout the world for internal and external treatment of wounds, sores, ulcers, and a wide variety of infections. In ancient days garlic was used to treat leprosy, smallpox, and other infectious diseases, and according to Mrs. Grieve, author of *A Modern Herbal*, historians revealed that during an outbreak of infectious fever in London during the last century, French priests who constantly used garlic remained healthy even though they were in contact with the worst cases. The English clergy, however, who also treated such patients but did not eat garlic, fell victim to the disease in many instances. Earlier, during the seventeenth century when the plague took the lives of thousands of French people, heavy garlic users were often spared the fate.

Russian researchers under the guidance of Professor B.P. Tokin investigated the old custom of wearing a clove of garlic around the neck for protection from infections and colds, and interestingly, found some merit for this old-wives' tale. While you might not be too keen on this type of jewelry, eating this pungent vegetable can protect and improve your health.

Numerous other plants also stimulate your natural defenses against infections, and the following basic herbal formula, consisting of herbs that have been found effective in the prevention and treatment of infectious diseases, help improve your natural immunity. Sweeten with a touch of honey, add one-third of a teaspoon of vitamin C powder and you have a potent and natural infection fighter that works.

Herbal Infection Fighter

1 oz. angelica root (*Angelica archangelica*)
1 oz. chaparral leaves (*Larrea divaricata*)
1 oz. echinacea root (*Echinacea angustifolia*)
1 oz. sassafras bark (*Sassafras officinalis*)
1 oz. thyme (*Thymus vulgaris*)
1 oz. white oak bark (*Quercus alba*)

Use: add 1 teaspoon of herbal mixture to 1 cup boiling-hot water, steep for 5 minutes, strain, and drink one to two cups per day.

SPECIAL TIPS FOR CONTROLLING NOSEBLEEDS

Children are frequently bothered by nosebleeds but adults are certainly not spared the trouble, and while this kind of hemorrhage can cause extreme blood loss, it is easily treated and prevented. Interestingly, a vitamin C deficiency is often found in individuals suffering from frequent nosebleeds, but supplementing the diet with ascorbic acid (pure vitamin C) alone is generally not enough to stop recurring nosebleeds. If, however, plenty of natural vitamin C (containing rosehips) is given to the patient, hemorrhaging can be prevented.

Bioflavonoids are the key to the prevention of nosebleeds, and sufficient amounts of bioflavonoids are easily obtained by eating fresh fruits, particularly oranges and other citrus fruits. The white skin underneath the orange peel is especially rich in bioflavonoids and eating this fibrous part is the simplest, cheapest, and most effective way of preventing nosebleeds. While oranges are considered one of the main sources of vitamin C and bioflavonoids, rosehips are even more nutritious, containing much vitamin A and other important nutrients. In comparison, 100 grams of rosehips contain 400 to 5,000 mg of vitamin C, while the same amount of oranges or lemons yields between 40 and 100 mg. For centuries, rosehip jam was Northern Europe's best, cheapest, and most easily available source of valuable nutrients which successfully strengthen and protect blood vessels from hemorrhaging. Homemade rosehip jam is truly one of Mother Nature's most nutritional delicacies.

The treatment of common nosebleeds is fairly simple. As soon as the bleeding starts get two ice packs. Sit or lie down, but keep your head up by putting a pillow under your head to prevent blood from rushing down to the broken blood vessels. Place one ice pack behind your neck and the other on your forehead. Place your fingers on the side of your nostrils, hold tight, and relax. Your nosebleed should stop quickly.

HOW TO DEAL WITH PLUGGED NASAL PASSAGES

The "stuffy nose syndrome" is frequently found in dry climates and becomes most bothersome during dry winter nights when the humidity in homes can be compared to that of the desert. The addition of a humidifier promptly helps, unless the problem is linked to allergies. In any case, increased humidity will bring relief.

Adding a drop of eucalyptus oil or menthol to specially equipped humidifiers quickly opens nasal passages. I, like many Europeans, have used this simple remedy for nasal problems. Of course, decades ago, before fancy humidifiers were available, people used to simmer water containing herbal oils on wood-burning stoves or mantelpieces to humidify the air with fragrant, deodorizing vapors. It works just as well.

A touch of Vicks Vapor Rub rubbed on the side of the nostril, under the chin, and on the forehead keeps nasal passages clear all night, and while Vicks is considered a modern product, it actually is a replica of an old-fashioned remedy. According to my books, lard mixed with a few drops of eucalyptus oil and menthol is the true forerunner of Vicks and similar products.

HELPING ALLERGIES AND SINUSITIS—
THE TRADITIONAL WAY

Sinusitis and allergies can be due to almost anything. You may be allergic to certain pollen in the air, foods, dust, even bacteria, or, attacks may be of emotional origin. Most likely, allergies and sinusitis have several causes, hence the treatment of sinus troubles and allergies is rarely simple, and is, in most cases, time consuming and frustrating. Though allergy testing is more sophisticated than ever, it rarely provides all the answers. Vaccination, though esteemed by the medical profession, provides no guarantee against attacks. The plain fact is that the usually long series of shots given to sinusitis and allergy sufferers may or may not help.

I have talked to many people who received "allergy shots" for years and who finally gave up on them. I also remember a few people who reported improvement, though in all of those cases, the emotional factor seemed to play a large part in their illnesses. When the underlying tension was removed, allergic reactions decreased and finally disappeared. Unfortunately, allergy victims have a difficult time admitting their inadequacy in handling stress. I recently talked with a man who suffered from excruciating allergy and sinusitis attacks that occurred frequently throughout the year. Although he vehemently denied the link to emotional problems, a violent sinusitis attack occurred as soon as he became upset with my inquiries. I mention this because it is necessary for the allergy victim to face the complexity of his problems. If he can't face his shortcomings or difficulties treatment cannot be successful.

I suspect that allergies are linked to hormonal changes. This happened to me during my last and otherwise very happy pregnancy. For some reason, I developed severe hayfever and sinusitis which were relieved only partially by supplements and by an otherwise highly nutritious diet.

Plugged nasal passages were relieved with camomile steam baths (see Chapter 1) to which I added a drop of eucalyptus oil. Inhaling these vapors helped more than any nasal spray and did not cause dependency or inflammation of mucous membranes, which can result in a vicious sinus infection.

For reasons unknown, hayfever attacks did not subside after the pregnancy, nor did they end with the pollen season. Instead, they remained bothersome and unpredictable companions all year around. When nasal drip and watering eyes replaced plugged nasal passages, the old-time remedy of licking table salt helped. To prevent or decrease the number of sinusitis attacks, I increased my daily vitamin C intake to 10 grams, and incidentally, scientists confirmed as early as 1940 that vitamin C is an effective antihistamine. In addition, I took 50,000 to 100,000 I.U. of vitamin A when needed, plus tremendous amounts of the B-vitamins (except PABA, which can intensify allergic reactions) and other nutrients. This nutritional regimen worked better than any antihistamine without causing drowsiness and other side effects, but again, it did not bring total relief.

During sinusitis attacks, I used acupressure to relieve congestion and stuffiness. All I did was to apply pressure to painful areas along the inner eyebrows until all or most of the local pain subsided. I must say, this simple self-treatment works exceptionally well and doesn't cost a dime.

Then one day my husband decided to try a series of acupuncture treatments. (I had received acupuncture treatments before, and though they had helped, they had not provided total relief.) As previously, needles were inserted around the sinuses, by the eyebrows, on top of the head, and other areas of my body, but this time two more were inserted in each small toe. Although I am not overly sensitive, these two needles caused extreme pain and I won't ever forget it. But surprisingly, after a few minutes all pain disappeared and I felt total relaxation. To make a long story short, a few of those treatments totally relieved my allergies, and only sometimes during the high pollen season do I notice a mild discomfort, which is easily controlled by an increased intake of the vitamins A, B, and C.

Just recently, I learned about some old German herbal tea formulas that prevent and ease hayfever attacks due to pollen. Apparently, these teas decrease your sensitivity to pollen and counteract hayfever and sinusitis attacks.

German Hayfever Teas

(eases hayfever attacks and sinusitis)

Formula 1

Mix 1 oz. eyebright (*Euphrasia officinalis*)
    1 oz. witch grass (*Agropyrum repens*)
    1 oz. wormwood (*Artemisia absinthium*)
    2 oz. masterwort (*Peucedanum ostruthium* or *Imperatoria ostruthium*)
    2 oz. pimpernel (*Pimpinella saxifraga*)
    3 oz. rue (*Ruta graveolens*)

Add 1 teaspoon herbal mixture to 2 cups cold water. Bring to boil and steep for 10 minutes. Strain and drink 1 cup before breakfast and another before dinner.

Formula 2

To be taken before pollen season to improve immunity.
Mix 1 oz. watercress (*Nasturtium officinale*)
    1 oz. coltsfoot (*Tussilago farfara*)
    1 oz. lungwort (*Pulmonaria officinalis*)
    1 oz. calendula (*Calendula officinalis*)
    1 oz. primrose (*Primula officinalis*)
    1 oz. cornflower (*Centaurea cyanus*)

Add 2 tablespoons herbal mixture to 2 cups cold water and let stand for 1 hour. Bring to boil and steep for 5 to 10 minutes. Strain and drink in small doses throughout the day.

NATURAL METHODS FOR BETTER EYESIGHT

Surgery on the eyes has become more sophisticated and artificial lenses are fancier than ever, but despite and perhaps because of all this, specialists are busier than ever treating eye conditions and the number of people depending on "crutches for the eye" has been increasingly steadily. More and more youngsters are wearing glasses or contact lenses, and although ophthalmologists realized as early as 1916 that glasses and other common medical treatments "are of but little avail" in improving nearsightedness, no attention is paid to prevention.

Nearsightedness, along with many other diseases of the eye, can be prevented but this won't happen unless parents and teachers are more aware of the causes, and consequently, of all the methods of prevention.

Just visit a modern classroom in any elementary school. Most likely, you will find children bent over paper work, little arms clutching desks and noses touching papers. Very rarely will you find a teacher who corrects poor writing habits which can be a major cause of nearsightedness, also called myopia. I've been to classrooms many times to observe children or to participate in some activity and each time I left feeling frustrated. The truth is, few teachers and parents care.

Just recently I talked with the father of a first-grader who within one year developed severe myopia. According to the distressed father, a previous eye examination taken the year before had revealed no eye damage, but within a few months problems appeared and nobody paid attention. By the time difficulties became obvious, severe myopia had developed and the child needed to be fitted with thick glasses. Of course, her teachers were aware of her extremely poor writing habits, but did not care enough to correct them.

Do you think this is an isolated case? Hardly. Add to this poor nutritional habits and you have a plausible explanation for the alarming increase in visual impairments among school children.

During my early school years, attention was paid to posture and I remember being tapped on the back many times because in those days everyone was expected to sit straight, especially while writing. Posture was considered important to total health including eyesight. Come to think of it, our eyesight was also checked regularly, yet not one of my elementary school classmates wore glasses. A coincidence? I don't think so.

Without normal eyesight every simple task becomes more difficult, though we hardly pay attention to these vital and complicated organs until problems arise. Our eyes deserve a lot of tender loving care, because without them we are quite helpless. Or, can you imagine a world of darkness? Wouldn't you miss that wonderful sensation of seeing?

The normal eye never *tries* to see. It automatically adjusts to whatever light conditions exist, and if it cannot see a particular object, rather than staring and straining itself, it shifts to another point. This indicates that the normal eye, like anything else, reacts to stress, and if given a chance, avoids it altogether.

Eyes with imperfect vision, however, have lost this ability. They strain themselves, for instance, by staring at hard-to-see points rather than shifting to other, easy-to-see objects and thus are subject to increased and damaging stress. This explains why people start out with minor eye problems and end up with major damage.

Relaxing the eyes is just as important as relaxing the mind. Moreover, one cannot rest the mind without resting the eyes and vice versa. Apparently, the health of the eye depends upon blood circulation and circulation is influenced by thought. Mental strain, for instance, can produce all sorts of eye problems. This is evidenced by the fact that many students end up with poor eyesight. On an average, blue-collar workers have better eyesight.

Interestingly, the relaxed eye instinctively focuses on a distant point and this phenomenon can be easily observed in a relaxing child. Before falling asleep, most young children stare at a fictitious, distant point, which indicates that the mind and eyes are relaxing.

While you may think that reading or watching TV is relaxing, it actually strains rather than relaxes the eyes, and if these activities replace needed rest periods, you are inviting vision problems.

Fortunately, defective eyesight can be corrected in its early stages and you don't need a physician to help you. All you have to do is to practice a few simple exercises each day, and once again, learn how to relax.

If you wear glasses, take them off. Choose a comfortable position in a room with a view, or better yet, go outside in a shady place. Place a book or cards with large and fine print at a distance from which you can barely read the large print, or better yet, get test cards as used by ophthalmologists for testing eyesight. These cards are ideal because they feature different size prints that can help you in your eye training. First find a distant point and relax while looking at it. Stare at it for as long as it feels comfortable, which may be a few seconds or several minutes, and quickly return to the large lettering in front of you. Repeat this exercise several times, eventually shifting to smaller and smaller print. When you start feeling tired, stop. Close your eyes and relax while thinking of something agreeable. You need to do this every day for several minutes.

I often tell people who are skeptical about this eye exercise program that during my last years of school I had been diagnosed as being near-sighted and had to wear glasses or else I would suffer from severe headaches. My father, who had lost part of his eyesight during a chemical accident, was very concerned and constantly urged me to use the above exercise program before problems became worse. Finally, after the excitement of wearing fancy glasses that gave me a real studious look had worn off, I decided to give it a try. Mother insisted on adding another old-fashioned remedy that has been used successfully to treat strained eyesight for centuries—carrot juice—one large glass every day, which incidentally, supplies approximately 50,000 I.U. of vitamin A.

Before the finals, I was able to shed the glasses, and today, nearly 20 years later, I enjoy perfect vision. It took some effort, but I suppose you get what you work for.

HEALTHY FOODS FOR HEALTHY EYES

Bad working habits as seen in students can induce a number of visual problems, but if coupled with bad nutritional habits, diseases of the eyes become more acute. As a matter of fact, severe nutritional deficiencies can induce a number of ailments, including blindness. Therefore, in countries such as India where diets are often grossly inadequate eye problems abound.

Good nutrition is vital to good eyesight and can prevent and actually improve visual problems. A healthy diet protects you from numerous diseases and has a profound effect on the eyes.

Long before vitamin A deficiencies were associated with diseases of the eyes, European folk healers "prescribed" carrot juice for the prevention and treatment of all sorts of eye problems with excellent results, and hundreds of years ago, long before vitamin A became a household word, babies were already spoon-fed mashed carrots and given carrot juice "to improve eyesight and resistance to disease." At times, eager mothers overdid this a bit and some babies turned yellow, but as soon as the carrots were withdrawn from the diet, the babies' color returned to a healthy pink.

One glass of carrot juice supplies approximately 50,000 I.U. of pro-vitamin A, or beta-carotene, which is water-soluble and can be excreted with the urine. This greatly reduces the risk of vitamin A overdoses.

Liver is another highly nutritious food that supplies an abundance of nutrients including vitamin A. One two-ounce slice of liver, for instance, supplies about 30,000 I.U. of vitamin A and one cup of cooked dandelion greens provides you with approximately 20,000 I.U. of this valuable vitamin.

The danger of vitamin A toxicity has been much publicized, and many people are afraid to take vitamin A supplements. In reality, food-induced vitamin A toxicity is extremely rare, especially in people who rely on water-soluble beta-carotene as found in vegetables.

The fact is, certain eye problems can be improved through a vitamin A-rich diet, and you don't need to fear toxicity—unless you indulge in polar bear liver, which has such an exceptionally high vitamin A content that it could cause temporary problems.

Of course, all nutrients are important to good health, and while vitamin A is considered to be essential to proper vision, the vitamins B, C, and E are equally important. Eyestrain as found in stressed individuals is often promptly relieved after sufficient amounts of the vitamin B-complex has been given to patients. An old-fashioned stress diet (see the "Antistress Diet Program," Chapter 6), which supplies good amounts of fresh fruit and vegetables, protein and some fat, is one of the best natural defenses against all eye diseases.

CORRECTING NIGHT BLINDNESS AND OTHER VISUAL PROBLEMS

Night blindness is as old as mankind. It was described in the Eber's papyrus in Egypt, a document over 3,500 years old, and this illness was, as writings reveal, successfully treated with ox liver. Hippocrates, the Greek physician, and other healers of ancient times such as the medicine men of Ruanda, Africa, also used ox liver to treat night blindness.

Night blindness is caused by a vitamin A deficiency, and those Newfoundland fisherman who eat plenty of codfish seldom encounter the problem. If, however, night blindness affects a Newfoundlander, codfish liver is prescribed which quickly restores normal night vision. Of course, cod liver oil has been used to treat eye problems for centuries.

Xerophthalmia, which literally means "dry eyes," is another eye disease clearly induced by a malnutrition. It is commonly observed among people when food is scarce, and is characterized by burning, itching, inflamed eyelids, and mucous in the corners of the eyes and the cornea. Though it is easily corrected nutritionally, neglecting treatment results in permanent blindness.

Protruding eyes are typical symptoms of a toxic thyroid, and nutritionists repeatedly reported that vitamin E supplementation not only improved the appearance of the eyes, but relieved hyperthyroidism, which is suspected to be caused, in part, by this very same deficiency.

Watering, burning, itching eyes; infections; blurred and dim vision; sandy eyelids and other abnormalities of the eyes can be alleviated by supplementing the diet with the vitamins A, E, and B-complex and are traditionally treated with a raw potato poultice that is applied directly to the eyes. This old-fashioned folk remedy eases strain, promotes healing, is extremely effective in relieving the feeling of "sand" in the eyes, and helps alleviate bloodshot eyes. Edgar Cayce, like many natural healers, was extremely fond of this simple treatment and recommended it with great success to many of his followers. Dr. Harold J. Reilly, founder and director of the famous Reilly Health Institute reports that he himself used potato poultices to relieve eyestrain and found them extremely effective.

Cayce's treatment plan for better eye care includes a highly nutritious diet, consisting of plenty of carrots, green peas and green beans, onions and beets, good amounts of citrus fruits, head and neck exercise, manipulation of the upper cervical area, and, of course, the above mentioned potato poultices.

Sea water relieves tired, sore eyes and, as Linda Clark said, "is surprisingly restful to the eye."[1] Although salt water at first stings the eyes, it irritates the eyes only temporarily. Since tears are salty as well, the eyes are used to this natural saline solution.

Salt water has long been used for minor eye problems, and while decades ago plain sea water was used as eye drops, *today's contaminated ocean water should not be used*. Use filtered sea water which may be found in health food stores. A few drops in each eye quickly relieve irritation.

During ancient days, herbal remedies provided relief from ocular problems, and red eyebright (*Euphrasia officinalis*) has been used as tincture, eyewash, or poultices by many cultures. Ancient healers such as Dioscurides and naturalists such as Theophrastus prescribed red eyebright with much success. Naturally, this all-time herbal remedy is still regarded among Europe's modern phytotherapists and health practitioners and continues to be a favorite homeopathic remedy. American herbalists are equally fond of red eyebright remedies, and a few years back, while interviewing Dr. Christopher, a well-known herbalist of Provo, Utah, I learned about many heartwarming success stories of people who successfully used eyebright.

---

[1] Used with permission of Devin-Adair Company. From *Handbook of Natural Remedies for Common Ailments*, by Linda Clark.

Certainly, I would be the last one to say that this herbal remedy is a panacea for eye diseases, but I can say that it is a valuable natural remedy that has helped many. Unfortunately, most American doctors show no interest in old-time remedies, even though many natural therapies have been around much longer than "orthodox" medicine. If we would combine traditional healing methods with modern medicine, wouldn't we all benefit?

SIMPLE REMEDIES FOR GLAUCOMA

Glaucoma, a common cause of blindness, is characterized by increased intraocular pressure which leads to pathological changes in the retina and the optic nerve. Although the disease has numerous causes, it can be separated into two categories: primary glaucoma, which is not preceded by other diseases of the eye; and secondary glaucoma, which typically follows some other ocular disease. Either case, however, seems to be related to stress and mental attitude. When the stress or underlying cause is removed symptoms often disappear, but unfortunately can reappear just as swiftly when stress or emotional problems return.

Glaucoma has also been linked to purely physical conditions such as defective circulation, sinus problems, allergies, diabetes, arteriosclerosis, disturbed pituitary function and the use of certain antispasmodic drugs or steroids such as cortisone. Altogether, glaucoma is a puzzling disease of varied origin, and medical treatment is seldom easy.

While there is much disagreement about treatment, nearly all ophthalmologists agree that caffeine, alcohol, and nicotine are detrimental to the patient. Since glaucoma seems to be associated with nutritional deficiencies, particularly a lack of the vitamins A, B, C, protein, calcium, magnesium and other minerals, glaucoma patients benefit from a supernutrition program. When generous amounts of the B-vitamins are supplemented improvement is often noticed. Of the B-vitamins, choline is particularly vital to the glaucoma patient because this nutrient is used by the body in the synthesis of acetylcholine, a neuro-transmitter of electrical impulses that is needed for proper nerve-muscle function. According to Dr. Carlton Fredericks, research demonstrates that choline, pantothenic acid, and manganese are especially important in the treatment of glaucoma and myasthenia gravis. Other well-known nutritionists, such as Ethel Maslansky of New York, indicate that niacin (another B-vitamin) and protein are equally important. In short, the typical glaucoma patient has great requirements for most nutrients. He should eat the best diet possible and avoid or counterbalance the harmful stressors in his life.

The renowned researchers Drs. E. Cheraskin and W.M. Ringsdorf also emphasize that it is necessary for glaucoma patients to avoid all stimulants including nicotine and to cut coffee and black tea consumption to one-half to one cup per day. (Beware of soft drinks; they are loaded with caffeine.) The patient's daily liquid intake, even in a hot climate, should never be excessive and fluid intake should be distributed throughout the day. Excessive TV viewing has to be restricted, though normal watching is permitted along with other ordinary activities such as reading, sewing, etc. Regular rest periods and relaxation techniques are also advisable.

Years ago, people like our old-fashioned family doctor recommended a stroll through the meadows. As ridiculous as it sounds, this ancient therapy actually relaxes the eyes. British researchers refer to this "treatment" as color therapy, and English studies demonstrate that the correct shades of green as found in nature actually lower intraocular pressure within ten minutes after exposure. While the British developed this simple remedy into a successful and sophisticated natural healing method that is used for many eye ailments with excellent results, a relaxing stroll through the meadows has to do for American patients, because color therapy is not approved by this country's medical profession.

A warm fennel eye bath and alternating red eyebright with camomile compresses are other folk treatments used by many European doctors. Although this simple herbal therapy is extremely successful in relieving ocular pressure, it has largely been replaced by modern drug therapy. Maybe because drug therapy is less time-consuming?

Again, the use of sea water, which has long been used to clear up inflammation and other eye problems, helps relieve ocular pressure. Linda Clark reports a man who had suffered from glaucoma for years and after the regular use of (filtered) sea water drops (found in health food stores) his ocular pressure returned to normal.

COMBINING OLD AND NEW TREATMENTS TO RELIEVE CATARACTS

The loss of transparency of the crystalline lens is known as cataract, and this is due to degenerative changes occurring in the lens proteins leading to opacity. Cataracts are often brought on by stress and are frequently seen in diabetics.

1. The Nutritional Approach

There are many types of cataracts and plenty of causes, and while stress, drugs, and radiation contribute to the disease, it is closely related to nutritional problems. Clinical researchers reported that some types of cataracts are due to calcium or other mineral deposits, while others have been linked to a vitamin C or protein deficiency or are caused by a fatty acid intolerance.

Dr. Roger J. Williams, a foremost authority on nutrition, states that a riboflavin (vitamin B2) deficiency produces cataracts in the eyes of experimental animals, and if the deficiency is not prolonged for too long, the cataracts disappear as soon as riboflavin is supplied. Although human cataracts have been successfully treated with riboflavin, not all cataracts respond to this treatment. Since it is, according to Dr. Williams, "reasonable to suppose that any of several nutritional deficiencies may be basic to the formation of cataracts,"[2] a supernutrition program is indicated, for experiments indicate that the correction of nutritional deficiencies can clear up the problem, but the diet must be high in protein, all B-vitamins, vitamins C and E, and other essential nutrients.

The proof that a faulty diet can cause cataracts can be seen in India and Pakistan where millions of young and middle-aged people suffer from cataracts. Apparently, their typical low-protein high-carbohydrate diet contributes to the disease. It is becoming more apparent that Eastern diets, many of which are becoming increasingly attractive to young Americans are not as healthy as people are led to believe. The macrobiotic diet, for example, can induce severe malnutrition and I have seen healthy, athletic people turn into malnourished and sick individuals after they had stayed on this diet for less than a year. Perhaps the many faddists who try these diets don't realize that certain celebrated dietary habits were dictated by economics rather than the body's nutritional needs.

2. Exercise

It is interesting that cataracts have stopped developing, even were reduced, through simple eye relaxation techniques. According to opthalmologists, many people who followed an eye exercise program (see this chapter) improved remarkably and escaped "inevitable" surgical procedures.

---

[2]Excerpt from *Nutrition in a Nutshell* by Roger Williams. Copyright © 1962 by Roger J. Williams. Reprinted by permission of Doubleday & Company, Inc.

3. Old-Time Natural Remedies

Traditional European therapies to improve cataracts include eye-bright tincture, camomile eyewash, and raw potato poultice, all of which benefit patients suffering from cataracts and other ocular disease. The English astrologer-physician Nicholas Culpeper who achieved fame in the early seventeenth century, was as fond of camomile eyewash and camomile eye drops as Sebastian Kneipp, who said that these remedies improve the condition and stimulate the healing process.

Castor oil, which was used by Cleopatra for beauty reasons, has been found to relieve all sorts of eye problems and continues to be used by those doctors dedicated to Edgar Cayce's teachings. Dr. Gladys of the A.R.E. (Association for Research and Enlightenment) Clinic of Phoenix, Arizona, recommends that castor oil should be rubbed around the eye, that is, inward from the outer edge of the eyelid and under the eye toward the nose, or be used as eye drops. According to Dr. Gladys, two drops in each eye before bedtime relieve the condition. Other therapists indicate that, if no improvement is noticed after one month, linseed oil (the one found in drugstores!) should be used instead. Apply one drop to each eye every night until an improvement is noticed.

Of course, Cayce often recommended head and neck exercises for eye problems, and Dr. Harold Reilly reports that Ruth Hagy Brod, co-author of *The Edgar Cayce Handbook for Better Health Through Drugless Therapy*, improved her eyesight with these simple rotation exercises. After she was told by an eye specialist that cataracts were developing in her eyes, she faithfully practiced Cayce's exercises, and within a short time the cataracts had partially dissolved.

The exercises are simple head and neck rotations and should be done several times a day.[3]

In her *Handbook of Natural Remedies For Common Ailments*, Linda Clark writes about another amazing natural remedy for cataracts—honey—and how it had healed the cataracts of a man and his horse after only a few applications. Apparently, all the man had done was to rub honey into the affected eyes, and though at first the honey stung and burned "like a thousand needles," it soon soothed and restored the eyesight of man and animal alike.

[3]From *The Edgar Cayce Handbook for Health Through Drugless Therapy* by Harold J. Reilly and Ruth Hagy Brod (Copyright © 1975 by Harold J. Reilly.) Used by permission of Macmillan Publishing Company.

Herbal Remedies for Better Eyesight

Camomile Eyewash

Add 1 teaspoon camomile flowers (*Matricaria chamomilla*) to 1 cup hot water. Steep for 3 to 5 minutes and strain using paper filter. Pour into eyecup and when lukewarm wash eyes, mornings and evenings.

Excellent for all eye problems especially inflammations, glaucoma, and cataracts.

Camomile Eyedrops

Add 1 tablespoon camomile flowers to ½ cup hot water and prepare like camomile eyewash. When cool, use eyedropper and add two drops in each eye several times per day.

Relieves inflammation and improves healing. Recommended for all eye problems including cataracts.

Camomile Poultice

Add ½ to 1 cup camomile flowers to 2 cups hot water and steep for 3 minutes. Strain and wrap flowers into washcloth. Wring out excess fluid and apply warm. Repeat if necessary.

Eyebright Eyewash

Steep 1 teaspoon of the fresh herb in 1 cup boiling-hot water for 5 minutes. Use like camomile eyewash. Recommended for all eye diseases.

Eyebright Eyedrops

Steep 1 heaping teaspoon of the fresh herb in ½ cup boiling-hot water for 5 minutes. Cool down and use like camomile eyedrops. Excellent for all eye ailments.

Fennel Eyewash

Add 1 teaspoon of powdered fennel seed (*Foeniculum vulgare*) to 1 cup boiling-hot water. Steep for 5 minutes and strain using paper filter. Pour into eyecup and when lukewarm wash eyes, mornings and evenings.

This treatment is for glaucoma and other ocular diseases. It is often alternated with camomile or red eyebright eyewash.

Raw Potato Poultice

Grate fresh potato (unskinned, if organic, otherwise remove skin), place between two layers of linen or gauze and place over closed eyelid for one half to one hour per day. Draws out impurities, relaxes and soothes eyes. Good for irritations, bloodshot eyes, inflammations, and other ocular problems.

****

References:

A.R.E. Medical Research Bulletin. Volume X, Number 4, December 1981.

Clark, Linda. *Handbook of Natural Remedies for Common Ailments.* Devin-Adair Co., 1976.

Davis, Adelle. *Let's Get Well.* Harcourt, Brace and World, Inc., 1965.

Fredericks, Carlton, Ph.D. *New & Complete Nutrition Handbook.* Major Books, 1976.

Goerz, Heinz. *Gesundheit durch Heilkraeuter.* W. Moeller Verlag, 1974.

Hutchens, Alma R. *Indian Herbalogy of North America.* Canada: Merco, 1969.

Lindt, Inge. *Naturheilkunde.* Buch und Zeit Verlag, 1977.

Lust, John B., N.D., D.B.M. *The Herb Book.* Bantam, 1974.

Pfeiffer, Carl, C., M.D., Ph.D. *Mental and Elemental Nutrients.* Keats, 1975.

Pierce, R.V., M.D. *The People's Common Sense Medical Advisor.* publisher unknown, 1921.

Reilly, Harold, Dr.; Brod, Ruth Hagy. *The Edgar Cayce Handbook for Health Through Drugless Therapy.* Macmillan, 1975.

Schauenberg, P.; Paris, F. *BLV Bestimmungsbuch.* BLV, 1978.

Simmonite-Culpeper. *Herbal Remedies.* Foulsham and Co., 1957.

Stage, Wolfgang, M.D. *Das Kneipp Taschenbuch.* Ullstein, 1968.

Steen, Edwin B., Ph.D.; Montague, Ashley, Ph.D. *Anatomy & Physiology.* Volume II, Barnes & Noble, 1959.

Williams, Roger J., Ph.D. *Nutrition in a Nutshell.* Doubleday, 1962.

10

Traditional Self-Help Remedies for Sports Injuries and Related Problems

YOU AND SPORTS

In my opinion, there are three kinds of people when it comes to sports: (1) the thoroughly physical type who is highly competitive; (2) the undecided type who enjoys exercise while he is doing it, but often has a hard time getting to it; and (3) the totally unphysical type who actually rejects and dislikes sports.

Type 1 remains fit throughout his life. He continues to ski on the expert slopes long after contemporaries have retired to less strenuous activities. The Type 1 personality never needs to be reminded of proper conditioning; instead, he constantly tries to improve, or at least keep up his physical capability. Such an individual starts scuba-diving, modern dance, racquetball, you name it, after retirement. He may roller-skate to his best friends' golden anniversary party, and climb Mount Everest when others have long enjoyed the rocking chair. In short, to him, testing and improving physical strength is one of the most important functions in life.

While Type 1 people remain physically fit throughout life, they occasionally "overdo it." Typical wear-and-tear injuries such as tennis elbow or bad knees are frequently found among them.

Type 2 individuals are more common. They often display considerable potential, but because they lack true competitiveness and are somewhat disinterested in physical activities, they don't exercise regularly. Therefore, these weekend athletes make up the millions of Monday-morning casualties seen in doctors' offices.

These people need proper conditioning to improve flexibility and muscle tone, or else sports may prove to be hazardous to their health.

The *Type 3* person may be an intellectual with a snobbish attitude towards sports, or he simply is lazy (too busy, he says) to be bothered. In either case, it is unlikely that he'll ever suffer from runners' aches or pains or muscle soreness, though it would be smart for him to read this chapter anyway—he may slip on the way to the refrigerator (library, office, store, etc.) and sprain his ankle.

PREVENTING SPORTS INJURIES

Most sports injuries need not occur. The startling fact is that most can be prevented using a simple common-sense approach. This means that you should let your body guide you through physical work, not vice versa. If you are a runner and your legs get sore, rest. If a throbbing headache bothers you before or during your weekend tennis match, don't try to be tough. Take care of yourself. The game can wait. If leg cramps prevent you from completing your thousand-meter swim, don't push yourself. Stop. Your body would not send you problem signals if everything were fine.

"When we feel good, look good, and are alert and productive," Tom Osler, author of "Avoiding All Injuries" (*Runner's World, The Complete Runner*, Avon, 1974) says, "our bodies will be adapting effectively to stresses (like running) which we place upon them. If we feel tired, pain and are washed out, we need rest, not stress."[1] Overtraining can be just as detrimental as if we train too little. The injury-free athlete works *with*, instead of against, his body.

EMERGENCY CARE FOR THE SERIOUSLY INJURED

Nobody in his right mind would question the fact that any major injury requires professional attention. Fractures, dislocated joints, or a major concussion, etc., call for emergency treatment (see Chapter 11), though not every injured individual has to end up in the doctor's office or hospital. I have seen nonmedical people take excellent care of dislocated joints at the scene of the accident and none of the injured athletes suffered from any side effects. On the contrary, since the injury was treated immediately and before swelling occurred, there was less damage

[1]Used with permission of Avon Books, The Hearst Corporation. "Avoiding All Injuries," by Tom Osler. From *Runner's World, The Complete Runner*, p. 101.

to the joint and ligaments. Generally, the more time that passes after such an injury, the more difficult, painful and even damaging corrective treatments are.

I speak from experience. At age 17, I dislocated my elbow while stepping off a train. To be more precise, I fell off the train. It took about 30 minutes to get to the hospital and another eternity to see the emergency doctor. By that time my whole arm was swollen to about twice its normal size and was extremely tender. The corrective adjustment was terribly painful and I won't ever forget it. The entire right arm was put in a cast, with which I lived through six long and hot summer weeks. It took corrective exercises to get the joint back to normal, but to this day my right arm is weaker and the elbow looks and feels strange. X-rays also indicate that this joint is not what it used to be.

About 20 years later I dislocated my shoulder while practicing judo. Our teacher (sensei) Mr. In Sun Hong, quickly applied emergency care and the joint was "put back" into place more quickly than I could have said "Mississippi." The procedure was relatively painless and I am ever so grateful that Mr. Hong reacted quickly and had the necessary skills to help. In the years since, I have seen high-ranking judo teachers apply expert emergency care to many injured competitors, including minor fractures, dislocated patellas (kneecaps), and other injuries that could have been far more traumatic.

Nowadays, chiropractors are becoming more recognized for their ability to deliver emergency help when it comes to musculoskeletal injuries. Like many other chiropractors my husband occasionally administers emergency care, and follow-up X-rays have never indicated healing problems. I mention this because just a short time back athletic programs discriminated against chiropractors. Thanks to the many athletes who simply chose to be treated by sports-minded chiropractic pioneers like Dr. Leroy Perry of California and others, D.C.s are now, and justifiably so, members of the Olympic and other such "medical" teams. These chiropractors do not only treat athletic injuries; they also stress prevention, the correction of structural problems, and educate athletes about proper self-treatment of minor injuries.

It is important to realize that the faster expert emergency care is delivered, the less traumatic the injury turns out to be. This is not to say, however, that an inexperienced spectator can take care of your injury. On the contrary, skill and knowledge is required to help the victim.

If someone seriously injures himself and nobody in the vicinity has the skill and knowledge to apply expert emergency care, call for help immediately or ask anybody to do so, and take the following precautions until professional help arrives:

1. If the victim is unconscious and bleeding from the mouth, turn his head gently to the side so that blood and mucus can drain from the corner of his mouth, and call for medical help. Lying quietly lessens the chance of severe hemorrhage. If you have some alcohol or lemon balm tincture handy, apply a few drops to the victim's temples.

   If the victim suffered a momentary loss of consciousness or cannot remember the injury, have him rest until emergency care has been administered. In some cases, the victim who has had a momentary loss of consciousness or a lack of memory of the event causing the injury, may insist that he feels good enough to continue his workout. Don't let him continue until you are certain that he does not display the following symptoms commonly related to head injuries, fractures and concussions:

   victim is dazed

   bleeding from mouth, nose, and/or ears

   pulse is rapid but weak

   pupils of eyes are unequal in size

   paralysis of one or more of the extremeties

   headache or dizziness

   double vision

   vomiting

   pallor

2. If a fracture is suspected don't move the patient. Have him rest and apply ice to the injured area. If possible, elevate injured area above heart level.

3. If a bandage must be applied, make sure it does not cut off circulation.

4. If swelling occurs, apply ice, *never* heat, and elevate the injured area above the level of the heart, if possible.

5. If a joint is dislocated, do not move it. If the victim dislocated a hand, arm, shoulder, or the jaw, safely transport him to the nearest doctor or hospital. If the hip is dislocated, immediately call an ambulance. Apply an ice bag or cold compress to any dislocated joint to reduce swelling.

WHEN AND HOW TO TAKE CARE
OF MINOR INJURIES

It cannot be overemphasized that every professional or weekend athlete should learn to take care of minor problems *before* they turn into major ones.

Minor injuries are those that do not require expert medical attention. If you fall and scrape your knees, suffer from a bloody nose, trip over a rock and mildly strain your ankle, or develop muscle cramps, you do not have to visit your hospital's emergency room. (Believe me, they have more serious cases to attend to.) Try simple old-fashioned remedies. They are effective, healthy, and easy-to-use and many of them are now approved and recognized as sound medical treatments.

TREATING STRAINS

A strain or muscle pull is a tear or rip on the muscle that may involve the hamstrings, calf muscles, or thigh muscles. Although painful, this injury is considered to be a minor problem, involving only a few muscle fibers. Generally, strains occur after a sudden muscle contraction that is followed by sharp pain, and in most cases, the injured area remains sore to the touch until healing occurs.

It is best to immediately apply ice and a compression bandage and later add arnica or marigold compresses or salve to speed up recovery.

QUICK SELF-HELP FOR SPRAINS

Sprains are one of the most common athletic injuries. They usually involve a twisting of a joint such as the ankle, knee, or shoulder, resulting in stretched or torn connective tissues. This often causes damage to ligaments, which connect bone to bone, and tendons, which connect muscle to bone. Blood seeping from torn capillaries into tissues can cause swelling and bruising depending on the severity of the injury.

It is best to elevate the injured joint or part of the body to a comfortable position that is preferably higher than the heart. Apply an ice bag or a cold compress for 30 minutes to reduce swelling and rest. After that, alternate ice packs with cold arnica compresses and keep resting.

To rule out the possibility of a fracture, you may want to call your doctor for an examination.

Cold Treatment

To apply cold, it is best to fill a plastic bag with crushed ice. Place a wet towel over injured area for 30 minutes, cover with ice bag, and leave on for 30 minutes. Remove and apply cold arnica compress. Repeat if necessary.

Arnica Compress

Add 1 tablespoon arnica tincture (*Tinctura arnica*) to 1 pint cold water and mix. Wet towel and apply to injured area.

Generally, pharmacies carry arnica tincture (often called arnica "extract"), but you can make your own by soaking 1 handful of fresh arnica flowers in 1 pint ethyl alcohol (70%) for two weeks.

Some time ago, a *Bestways* reader required information regarding arnica "fluid." I answered his questions and soon received a call from the reader, who incidentally lives in Denver. This man uses arnica tincture for his race horses because, "nothing heals bruises, strains, and sprains as quickly as this old-time remedy."

SIMPLE EUROPEAN REMEDIES PREVENT AND RELIEVE MUSCLE SORENESS AND OTHER ATHLETIC INJURIES

Repeated injuries are common among athletes, yet according to athletically-minded doctors like my husband and his partner Dr. Steven R. Campbell, they can be prevented. Apply heat to previously injured areas *before* your regular warm-up and training session, they say, and you will help avoid repeated injuries.

Regular exercise is the best insurance against muscle soreness. For example, if you are a distance runner just starting a weight-lifting program there is a good chance that your biceps and other previously neglected muscle tissues will react to the new muscle training and become sore.

You can prevent this painful stage by starting an exercise program that helps to gradually develop muscle strength, or, after you have over-exercised and expect soreness, soak in a hot tub or bath. Use juniper (*Juniperus communis* or *J. oxycedrus*) berries or young twigs, lemon balm (*Melissa officinalis*), and/or marigold (*Calendula officinalis*) flowers and leaves as bath additives to relax overworked, tense muscles. This simple precaution does prevent and relieve the worst muscle pain.

In Austria and Germany, the marigold herb, which has long been used to successfully relieve muscle soreness, sprains and strains, sores, bruises, and boils, is making a comeback.

Sebastian Kneipp was fond of this herb and used it for external injuries with great success. Today, European cancer specialists are beginning to substantiate that marigold tincture does not only aid external injuries and improve wound healing—it also aids certain cancers. Famous European medical doctors like Drs. Bohn, Staeger, and Halenser are now recognizing this old-time remedy as an important cancer therapy. Fresh marigold juice, these authorities say, does not only improve general wound healing; it can combat skin cancer.

Tincture and salve are easily prepared and are a must for anybody's medicine cabinet.

Preparation of Marigold Remedies

Bath additive: Add 2 handfuls of fresh or three ounces of dried herb to 1–2 quarts of hot water. Steep for 20 minutes, strain, and add liquid to bath water. Wrap strained herb into linen sack and hang into tub.

Tincture: Soak a handful of flowers in 1 quart brandy and store in the sun or a warm place for two weeks. Strain. To use, dilute with distilled water. (Note: marigold tincture is not as strong as arnica tincture and is especially useful for treating children and sensitive individuals.)

Salve: Mix 1–2 teaspoons fresh juice with 1 oz. lard or add two handfuls of fresh cut flowers and leaves to ½ pound of hot lard. Mix, remove from heat, and let stand overnight. Heat up again, strain, and fill jar with mixture.

FOLK HEALERS' REMEDY FOR BRUISES

While arnica tincture and marigold preparations are excellent herbal remedies for bruises, I was recently reminded of two excellent folk remedies that truly, and for a good reason, originated in Grandma's kitchen.

A *Bestways* reader wrote the following letter:

Dear Eleonore:

I am 17 and love the sport of boxing, but Mother is horrified when I come home with bruises. Last week, I got a black eye and Grandma told me to apply raw beefsteak. Well, I did and it worked, meaning it (the black eye) healed a lot quicker than normally. My question: how can raw meat help? I'd like to tell my friends about it, but I'm afraid I'll sound like a fool.

Randy S., San Antonio, TX

Here is my reply:

Dear Randy:

It's the potassium in the meat that does the job, however, since you seem to be in the market for bruises and black eyes, I suggest you try raw potato poultices instead. They are a lot cheaper and more effective.

Freshly grate a raw potato, apply to the bruised area, and leave on for 15 minutes or as long as it feels comfortable.

Potatoes are the richest natural source of potassium chloride, the most effective of all potassium compounds when it comes to healing bruises.

Enjoy the sport and tell Mother there are worse problems than bruises (for example, drugs and booze), and start moving away faster from those punches.

IMPROVING LOW BACK PAIN

Many athletes, dancers included, are afflicted with low back pain which often is the result of direct injury, inherent weakness, or simple abuse. While rest may be indicated, chiropractic treatment can certainly help the athlete recover more quickly. Vitamin C has been found to prevent and aid low back pain. 500 mg to 10 grams per day of this vitamin has been "prescribed" to improve low back pain problems with astonishing results. In addition, an overall improvement in athletes' nutritional status reportedly helped to alleviate pain. Generally, when the diet supplies adequate amounts of protein, calcium, magnesium, and vitamins D and C, backaches gradually disappear, and as an extra bonus, the athlete often experiences fewer fractures.

Chronic pain responds remarkably well to hot linseed poultices and massages using St. Johnswort oil. Acute pain, however, should *never* be treated with heat. Apply ice and go to see a chiropractor.

Linseed Poultice for Chronic Pain

Soak 1 cup of linseeds in cold water overnight. Bring to boil and apply as hot as is tolerable. Linseeds can be reheated a few times.

St. Johnswort Massage Oil Helps Relieve Pain

Add fresh St. Johnswort flowers (*Hypericum perforatum*) to jar and cover with olive oil. Tightly close jar and store in warm place or in the sun for three to five weeks (the oil should have turned red by then) and strain. Pour oil into a dark-colored glass jar and store in a dark, cool area, but don't refrigerate.

TAKING CARE OF TORN CARTILAGE

A cartilage, usually held in place by ligaments, is a type of connective tissue that, among other functions, allows smooth motion of a joint. A direct blow to a joint such as the knee or elbow can dislodge or twist the cartilage, resulting in a tear that can cause severe pain and loss of motion.

Plenty of vitamin C and a diet high in protein improves healing and can prevent surgery. Amino acids such as methionine and vitamin E are essential to proper healing of torn cartilage, including damaged or degenerative discs.

Folk healers have long used comfrey (*Symphytum officinale*) to aid all sorts of athletic injuries including damaged cartilage, and the famous Austrian herbalist Maria Treben reports that comfrey (German: Beinwell or Beinwurz) is extremely helpful for all musculoskeletal injuries and certainly speeds up the healing process. Like many European and American herbalists, Maria Treben considers comfrey one of the most useful medicinal herbs, and in case of injury recommends two to four cups of comfrey tea per day plus the application of comfrey poultices.

Comfrey Tea for Better Healing

Add two teaspoons of cut rootstock to 1 cup cold water and soak overnight or add 1 teaspoon cut leaves to 1 cup hot water and steep for 5 minutes. Strain, and drink 2–4 cups throughout the day.

Comfrey Poultice to Speed Up Recovery

Add hot water and a few drops of olive oil to dried, chopped rootstock or rootstock powder until a thick mash is formed. Spread on linen cloth and apply to injured area. Renew every two to four hours. Also good for tennis elbow and other athletic injuries.

COPING WITH LEG CRAMPS

Like my parents and brothers, I am a good swimmer, and while I, too, was considered "a potential winner," reality proved otherwise.

The reality was leg cramps. During my teenage years I entered competitive swimming, but whenever I tried extra hard, incapacitating muscle spasms ended the dream. It was agony and nobody understood the problem or provided the slightest clue on how to control the cramps.

Years later, while taking calcium and magnesium to combat an allergy problem, the leg cramps, which had continued to bother me, disappeared. Calcium and magnesium had been the missing link.

In the years since, I have often recommended calcium and/or magnesium to prevent or relieve leg cramps and similar muscle spasms, and the results always spoke for themselves. Although magnesium is generally not associated with spastic conditions, a deficiency is associated with daytime spasms, while a lack of calcium most often is the cause of night cramps.

The most interesting case was that of a friend who, when nervous, suffered from an involuntary twitch of the eye. After he started taking a calcium/magnesium supplement the problem lessened and soon disappeared.

Leg cramps, however, may have a number of causes, among them a vitamin B-6 deficiency and an increased need for vegetable oils and the vitamins E and C which help improve circulation.

A muscle spasm, also called a "charley horse," can be relieved quickly by careful stretching exercises, though the athlete must be careful or injury may occur. After the spasm has been relieved, rest and apply a marigold compress and follow with a gentle massage using marigold salve.

Strangely enough, leg cramps often occur at night and may afflict the leg, calf, or foot. To relieve the spasm, turn on your back and slowly try to point the toes towards the ceiling. If this does not help, get up, take a magnesium supplement, and walk around or soak in a warm tub of water. Drink a cup of the following antispasmodic tea, which helps relieve and prevent cramps and spasms.

Antispasmodic Tea

Mix:

1 oz. camomile flowers (*Matricaria chamomilla*)
1 oz. cinquefoil (*Potentilla anserina*)
1 oz. lemon balm (*Melissa officinalis*)
1 oz. hops (*Humulus lupulus*)
½ oz. valerian (*Valeriana officinalis*)

Add 1 teaspoon of the herbal mixture to 1 cup hot water, steep 3 minutes, strain, and drink.

OVERCOMING RUNNERS' ACHES AND PAINS

During my childhood, doctors examined and evaluated patients' feet. That may sound strange nowadays, but then the feet were considered to be an important part of your body and doctors commonly prescribed simple supports to correct structural problems.

Somewhere along the line, runners picked up the idea that simple shoe modifications, which support imperfect feet, can eliminate certain runners' problems. Athletes learned to apply a few basic principles—and found relief from troubles with arches or muscles, achilles tendinitis, even shin splints.

Bill Weigle, Olympic team member and AAU champion of the 50 kilometer race in 1972, says that in 1971 shin splints made training almost impossible. After it was discovered that weak arches and a leg that was about one-half an inch shorter than the other caused all that agony, corrective supports not only eliminated the problems but helped improve his performance.

According to Tom Knott, a well-known runner, arch supports can be made easily. He actually recommends cutting little rubber "cookies" to fit your arches. "I use a piece of sponge rubber that does not compress easily," he said, "and carve it to shape. I stick them in each pair of shoes with two-sided tape. If not stuck down, they slip and end up under my heel, especially when running. If anyone," he said, "is having the slightest bit of trouble with achilles tendons, arches, or muscles in the back of the legs, the cookie supports are worth trying. I know of no way they can hurt, and they certainly have helped me."

Tendinitis is the runner's worst nightmare, and though heat and rest are always effective, a week to ten days may be required before the athlete can resume fully active training. Among European athletes and health care providers, hot mud applications or ultrasound therapy are considered the most effective treatments that can, if properly used, shorten recovery time considerably.

TRADITIONAL REMEDIES FOR SENSIBLE FOOT CARE

"Considering that the foot bears the entire weight of the body 1,500 times while walking a mile, it is indeed a wonder that people get about at all, let alone participate in marathons," says Thomas B. Quigley, M.D. How true that is, though we all know getting around is not always easy.

A hot foot bath is an excellent remedy for tired, sore, and/or burning feet and it becomes a heavenly palliative after the addition of specific natural ingredients. Cold foot baths feel wonderful on hot summer days and promote circulation and even relieve nosebleeds. Alternating between cold and hot (one to two minutes in the hot water; and one-half to one minute in the cold), relieves tired and sore feet, promotes circulation, aids high blood pressure, relieves chronically cold feet, prevents varicose veins, and even colds.

Old-Time Healing Foot Baths

Athlete's foot:

Marigold (*Calendula officinalis*). Add 3–4 oz. to 1 pint hot water, steep for 10 minutes and strain.

Thyme (*Thymus vulgaris*). Use: see marigold.

Bruises:

Arnica (*Arnica montana*). Steep 2–3 oz. in pint hot water for 5 minutes and strain.

Lavender (*Lavandula vera, L. officinalis*). See arnica.

Marigold (see directions above).

Rosemary (*Rosmarinus officinalis*). Add 1 cup leaves to 1 pint hot water and steep for 10 minutes. Strain and add decoction to water.

Thyme (*Thymus vulgaris*). Steep 1 to 2 oz. in 1 pint of boiling-hot water for 10 minutes. Strain and add decoction to tub water.

Burning, to relieve:

Bran. Add 3–4 oz. bran to 1 quart cold water, bring to boil, and steep for 5 minutes. Strain.

Circulation, to improve:

Mustard seed (*Brassica nigra*). Put ½ lb. ground mustard seed into linen sack and add to boiling-hot water. Boil for 30 minutes. Add decoction to footbath.

Rosemary. (See directions above.)

Shave grass (*Equisetum arvense*). Boil 3 oz. in 1 qt. water for 10 minutes and strain.

Sweet flag root (*Acorus calamus*). Add 3 oz. to 1 qt. cold water and let soak for 2 hours or more. Bring to boil and steep for 10 minutes. Strain.

Eczema:

Rosemary (see directions above) plus 1 tablespoon borax.

Frostbites:

Walnut leaves (*Juglans regia*). Use fresh ones if possible. Add 1 handful cut leaves to 1 pint boiling-hot water and steep for 10 minutes. Strain.

Inflammation:

Camomile (*Matricaria chamomilla*). Add 1 cup flowers to 1 pint hot water and steep for 10 minutes. Strain.

Sores:

Camomile.
Oak bark (*Quercus alba, Q. rubra, Q. tinctoria*). Steep 1 handful bark in 1 pint water for 30 minutes and strain.

Sprains:

Arnica.
Marigold.
Thyme.

Stimulating:

Add 1 lb. fresh pine cones or twigs to 1 qt. cold water and soak overnight. Boil for 2 hours and strain.

Strains:

Arnica.
Marigold.
Thyme.

Swellings:

Comfrey (*Symphytum officinalis*). Steep 2–3 oz. in 1 pint hot water for 5 minutes and strain.
Arnica.
Marigold.
Thyme.

Sweating, excessive:

Oat straw (*Avena sativa*). Add 1 lb. oat straw to 1 qt. cold water, boil for 30 minutes and strain.
Shave grass.
Oak bark.
Walnut leaves. Add 1–3 oz. leaves to 1 pint water. Bring to boil and steep for 10 minutes. Strain.
Also lightly dust the soles of your shoes with flowers of sulfur. This old-fashioned, popular European remedy can work wonders.

Wounds:

As an antiseptic: Thyme.
To promote healing: Arnica (*Arnica montana*). Steep 1 oz. in pint hot water for 10 minutes and strain.
Camomile.
Comfrey.
Shave grass.
For infectious wounds: Walnut leaves.

USEFUL REMEDIES THAT REMOVE CALLUSES, CORNS AND BUNIONS

These common foot problems are the result of irritation. Take a celandine (*Chelidonium majus*) footbath every morning and night and gently remove excess skin. In the mornings massage area with vitamin E oil; in the evenings apply fresh celandine juice and within a short time your feet should feel like new.

Celandine Foot Bath

Add 1 handful celandine herb to 1 pint hot water and steep for 30 minutes. Strain and add to bath.

Celandine Juice

Clean fresh herb and place in juicer (centrifuge type works well). Apply thinly to calluses and bunions and gently dab on corns, but no more than two to three times daily. This treatment is also good for warts.

SIMPLE TREATMENT FOR FROSTBITES

Just before frostbite occurs the victim's skin may be flushed, and as the freezing progresses turn white or gray-yellow. The patient may or may not complain about pain.

Do not apply snow. Immediately cover the frozen area with a warm blanket, clothes, or your warm hand, but do not apply a heated blanket or pad or a hot-water bottle. Do not rub overexposed areas or place the patient near a stove because excessive heat can cause tissue damage. Instead, have the patient drink hot tea with lemon and have him take a warm bath not exceeding 95 degrees Fahrenheit. Add shave grass (*Equisetum arvense*) decoction to bath water, or oak bark decoction if skin is chapped and bleeding. After the bath, gently rub marigold salve onto affected areas and encourage patient to exercise affected parts.

****

References:

"Athletic Injuries." *Current Health 2*, Sept. 1978.

Cheraskin, E., M.D.; Ringsdorf, W.M., Jr., D.M.D. *Predictive Medicine.* Keats, 1973.

Clark, Linda. *Handbook of Natural Remedies for Common Ailments.* Devin-Adair, 1976.

Editors of Runner's World Magazine. *The Complete Runner.* Avon, 1974.

Furlenmaier, M., M.D. *Wunderwelt der Heilpflanzen.* Germany: Rheingauer Verlag, 1978.

Goerz, Heinz. *Gesundheit durch Heilkraeuter.* Germany: W. Moeller, 1974.

Lindt, Inge. *Naturheilkunde.* Germany: Buch und Zeit, 1977.

Lust, John B. *The Herb Book.* Bantam, 1974.

Miller, Lois Mattox; Thompson, Susan W. *Handbook of First Aid.* Reader's Digest Assn., 1975.

Reilly, Harold J.; Brod, Ruth Hagy. *The Edgar Cayce Handbook for Health Through Drugless Therapy.* New York: Macmillan, 1975.

Schauenberg, P.; Paris, F. *BLV Bestimmungsbuch.* Germany: BLV, 1978.

Steen, Edwin, Ph.D.; Montagu, Ashley, Ph.D. *Anatomy and Physiology.* Volume 1. Barnes & Noble, 1959.

Strauss, R.H., M.D. *Sports Medicine and Physiology.* Saunders, 1979.

Thompson, William A.R., M.D. *Heilpflanzen und ihre Heilkraefte.* Germany: Lingen, 1978.

Treben, Maria. *Gesundheit aus der Hausapotheke.* Austria: Ennsthaler, 1980.

11

Golden Remedies
for "Incurable" Diseases

CANCER—WHAT CAUSES IT?

Diseases caused by the environment can be successfully fought by changing the environment. Louis Pasteur, on his deathbed, said, "The microbe is nothing. The soil (environment in which it grows) is everything," and after decades of ignoring environmental factors, scientists are beginning to recognize environmental causes of cancer.

One of the reasons for this growing recognition is the climbing rate of lung cancer in American women. Dr. Arthur Holleb, senior vice-president for medical affairs of the American Cancer Society (ACS), predicted that lung cancer would be the leading killer by 1985.

Despite the ACS's anti-smoking campaign, cigarette smoking causes an estimated 100,000 cancer deaths each year. The sober fact is that tobacco is responsible for 30 percent of current cancer deaths. Presently, most of these cancer victims are men, but this trend is quickly changing. More women are becoming victims.

Nutritional factors are linked to a number of cancers because diet affects the formation and transport of carcinogens (cancer-causing agents). A low-fiber diet, for instance, slows down elimination, thus promoting the formation of potent carcinogens. Dr. David Reuben, author of *The Save Your Life Diet*, says that Americans who are on a lifelong low-roughage diet are probably converting their own harmless bile acids into two awesome cancer-causing chemicals, apcholic acid and 3-methyl-cholantrene, within their own large intestines. The present estimate is that up to 70 percent of all cancers are caused nutritionally.

Two British epidemiologists, Sir Richard Doll and Richard Peto of

Oxford University, have estimated that between 75 and 80 percent of all American cancer deaths could be prevented. Presently, cancer causes are estimated as follows:

Tobacco—30%

Diet—10-70%

Infection—10%

Sexual factors, including multiple partners, childbirth, and pregnancy—7%

Occupation—4%

Alcohol—3%

(Recent studies indicate that alcohol-induced cancers are greater than anticipated, thus this figure could be much greater.)

Geographical location, including radiation exposure from sun and space—3%

Environmental pollution—2%

Medicine, medical treatment, including X-rays—1%

Food additives—1%

Industrial products—1%

Irving J. Selikoff, director of the Environmental Sciences Laboratory at Mt. Sinai Hospital in New York is less conservative. He predicts that 95% of all cancers are caused by environmental factors.

REDUCING THE CANCER RISK

Personal environment (including ethnic eating habits), water supply, and employment are all linked to cancer deaths, the Environmental Protection Agency reported. The study showed a cancer mortality rate of 20 percent above the national average for the area from New York City to Philadelphia, and a 10 percent increase for the 49 counties studied in New Jersey, New York, Pennsylvania, Connecticut and Delaware. According to the reports, a high incidence of cancer is linked to ethnic lifestyles. For example, the rate of stomach cancer is high among the Polish, while breast cancer causes a high mortality rate among Italians.

Changing genetic links may be impossible, improving cancer risks is not. As my mother says, "If you want miracles, perform them."

You alone may be unable to reduce pollution or improve the overall quality of your water, but you do have some political impact. Remember that the next time you vote.

Occupational hazards can be reduced or avoided, and more and more companies are upgrading existing standards. Don't let your boss forget his or her responsibilities.

Avoid stress, another strong link to cancer. Dr. Paul Roesch, internist and clinical professor of medicine at New York Medical College, is convinced that stress causes cancer. Modern research, he says, is slowly catching up with the old-fashioned wisdom of centuries, which long has held that emotional trauma caused cancer. Stress, Dr. Roesch states, inhibits our immune system, and while every individual develops millions of cancer cells many times during his life, a healthy immune system destroys these invaders. The theory that those people who "put up a good fight" and basically believe in recovery are those who have the best survival rate, is becoming increasingly accepted among psychologists and stress researchers.

Nutritional factors prevent or contribute to cancer. The old saying, "You are what you eat" still stands. Recently, the National Academy of Sciences stated in its report, "Diet, Nutrition and Cancer," that dietary habits increase or lower risk of cancer. Specific vegetables such as those from the cruciferous family—cabbage, broccoli, cauliflower, kale, brussel sprouts—are definitely associated with a *reduced* incidence of stomach, colon, and rectal cancer. A possible link between a high-protein intake and cancer was also suggested.

It is my humble opinion that diseases such as cancer are even more closely tied to dietary habits, and that the doctor of the future will be more of a nutritionist than a surgeon or pharmaceutical dispenser.

The healing force of certain foods may be largely overlooked but I am certain it won't be denied forever. Unsweetened juices of beets, carrots, blackberries, blueberries, and elderberries, for instance, are part of Europe's most effective cancer diets. Berries are high in benzaldehyde (a natural cancer-fighter that is part of laetrile), vitamin C, and anthocyan, a natural color pigment Europeans believe to be effective in the fight against cancer. Carrots and beets, however, supply ample amounts of beta-carotene (provitamin A), the nutrient that has been found to block the formation of cancer.

A recent cancer study from England involving 16,000 men measured the vitamin A (retinol) levels in serum and the results revealed that the increased risk of cancer is associated with low vitamin A levels.

The National Cancer Institute is beginning to investigate the nutritional connection. One study uses medical doctors as guinea pigs (what a change), and every day now, some 17,000 healthy middle-aged doctors across the country swallow a capsule that may contain vitamin A (beta-carotene), or be a dummy pill. This study, spanning a total of five years, intends to find out whether vitamin A protects against cancer. The only drawback is, in my opinion, that the individual vitamin A intake, which is the equivalent to three carrots a day, may be too low to produce significant results. If that is the case, vitamin A may be dismissed as ineffective, and consequently, many cancer patients would be discouraged from using it.

The fact is, at least 20 different population studies in the United States and seven other countries indicate that people who eat higher-than-average amounts of carrots and green, leafy vegetables (for most people, the main source of beta-carotene) have lower-than-average cancer rates.

The toxicity of excessive vitamin A has been widely publicized. People are actually scared to take this nutrient, even though studies conducted by the United States National Nutrition Survey present evidence that the American population shows a substantial vitamin A deficiency. Thirty-three percent of our children under six years of age are deficient in this valuable nutrient. This being the case, how can we expect a drop in cancer rate among children?

Exactly how much vitamin A is too much is disputed. One thing is certain, the minimum daily requirement of 1,500 to 4,500 I.U. per day is not enough, and the scare tactics are ridiculously misleading. Vitamin A is not nearly as dangerous as aspirin. I have yet to see a vitamin A toxicity, and I have worked with people who have taken 100,000 I.U. daily for one week or more.

Our daughter has taken between 10,000 and 30,000 I.U. ever since she was able to swallow nutritional supplements, and before that she ate mashed liver, carrots, and other vitamin A-rich foods regularly without ever developing xanthosis, a yellow discoloration of the skin due to excessive accumulation of carotene (precursor of vitamin A) in the body. On occasion, she has taken up to 60,000 I.U. daily for a short time, without experiencing any ill effects. During a bout with pneumonia, I have taken more than 100,000 I.U. for several weeks without experiencing toxic effects. On the contrary, vitamin A definitely shortened convalescence. Generally speaking, it is my experience that between 10,000 and 30,000 I.U. of vitamin A can be taken indefinitely by the average adult without causing any harm, and 50,000 to 100,000 I.U. can be taken for a short period of time, depending on the case.

For the average school-age child, 10,000 to 20,000 I.U. of vitamin

A per day pose no danger. During illness, more may be given temporarily without problems, depending on the child's body size.

To assure you that the values outlined here are, indeed, conservative, let me tell you about the Dutch crew who caught a 6½-foot halibut in the North Atlantic of Norway. One crewman ate two-thirds of a pound of the liver, containing approximately 30 *million* units of vitamin A. He developed severe frontal headaches, nausea, vomiting, abnormal gait, and red and swollen skin, with severe loss of the top layers of his skin, but he recuperated.

Certainly, other people have experienced toxicity after ingesting considerably less vitamin A, but the danger of dying from vitamin A toxicity is minute. Your chances of dying from a drug overdose or drug reaction are much greater, indeed.

Early signs of vitamin A poisoning are red discoloration of the gums, craving for food, or lack of appetite, itchy skin and/or skin peeling, muscle stiffness, bursitis, and headaches from increased intracranial pressure. Symptoms of acute toxicity are nausea, vomiting, vertigo, irritability, drowsiness, and in severe cases, seizures, and eventually, coma. In case any of these toxic symptoms appear, immediate cessation of vitamin A intake promptly provides relief.

Dr. Linus Pauling's often ridiculed theory that ascorbic acid (vitamin C) is beneficial in preventing and treating cancer has been confirmed by a group of researchers at Children's Hospital in Los Angeles. Drs. William F. Benedict and Peter A. Jones, who conducted animal studies, reported that low doses of vitamin C prevented or reversed cell transformation, which normally occurs after animal tissues are exposed to carcinogenic agents. According to the scientists, vitamin C could be added as late as 23 days after exposure and still inhibit cancer formation.

Now, it is true that animal studies don't represent human experiments. Thus, Dr. Pauling, who does not have a clinic but cooperates with the noted Scottish researcher and surgeon Dr. Ewan Cameron, began studying vitamin C almost 15 years ago in hospitals in Scotland and found that the life expectancy of terminally ill patients who receive 10 grams of vitamin C per day is seven times greater than that of other terminally ill patients who have not received the supplement.

Selenium, like vitamins C and E, is an effective antioxidant that helps prevent chromosome breakage in tissue culture. Damaged chromosomes, Dr. Carl C. Pfeiffer says, cause not only birth defects but can also result in cancer. Selenium increases the effectiveness of vitamin E and protects against the toxic effects of pollutants such as cadmium. Low selenium levels are associated with cancer.

It has long been known that certain foods offer protection from cancer. In 1950, Dr. Sugiura, a Japanese-American biochemist at the Sloan-Kettering Institute for Cancer Research, tested brewer's yeast and liver. During the experiment laboratory rats were fed varying amounts of these highly nutritious foods and then were inoculated with a powerful cancer-causing chemical. All animals who had received the normal, quite nutritious diet soon came down with cancer, but those rats whose diet consisted of 15% brewer's yeast showed no signs of cancer whatsoever. Liver supplementation produced even more startling results. Only 10% of the animals' diets needed to consist of liver to totally protect them from cancer. Dr. Sugiura's results were published in the Journal of Nutrition on July 10, 1951—and ignored by conventional cancer researchers ever since.

Unfortunately, other important studies were equally ignored. In 1957, scientists at Western Reserve University demonstrated that rats inoculated with a substance isolated from garlic demonstrated improved resistance to carcinogens.

At the University of Nebraska's Epping Cancer Institute, researchers found that small amounts of yogurt added to the diets of laboratory animals improved their resistance to induced cancer.

European cancer specialists insist that a diet high in fats and simple carbohydrates (sugar, white flour, etc.) leads to cancer, particularly stomach cancer. According to Dr. H.O. Kleine, M.D., German cancer specialist, this is evident by the high rate of stomach cancer among Swedes and Polish people who are known to eat diets high in fats. The British, however, who have a moderate intake of fats, have one-third that cancer rate.

How much more evidence do you need before you fight your own war against cancer?

LOOKING AT AN OLD-WIVES' TALE

How I remember the embarrassing mother-daughter talks about how "the loose girls have to pay for their sins eventually," followed by the not-so-discreet hints, "Look at so-and-so. She's got cancer ... (of the unspeakable)." Of course, when these talks were somewhat focused on me and other girls some twenty or thirty years ago, only mothers made these connections.

So it was surprising to hear the same lecture all over again, only this time from a well-known medical doctor who backed up Mother's theory with statistics.

According to Dr. Mendelsohn, risk factors for vaginal cancer are: (1) the pill, (2) the IUD, and (3) sexual intercourse with multiple partners. While sexual activity may lead to vaginal cancer, it does not cause breast cancer. Nuns have no vaginal cancer, but because of failure to conceive and failure to breast-feed, have a high rate of breast cancer. Other factors causing breast cancer are the pill and postmenopausal hormones.

Despite medical advancement, what Mother insisted on years ago still holds up, "When it comes to sex, there are no simple answers. Moderation is your best policy." Darn it.

NATURAL CANCER THERAPIES

Despite efforts to suppress increasing evidence that natural therapies are useful in combating cancer, these unconventional forms of cancer treatments become more visible each year.

Which one is the most promising? You will have to decide for yourself, for if you strongly believe in a certain therapy, stress researchers say, your chances of survival are considerably greater.

Nutrition seems to be the most promising natural method of prevention and treatment, and many diets are publicized, each one slightly different from the other. I find it difficult to say which one is superior to the other, though the most widely known and researched diet is the Gerson therapy which includes a strict detoxification program. This diet, like most cancer diets, is based on raw organic fruits and vegetables and juices. It largely eliminates meat and forbids all processed foods. Canned, salted, pickled, prepared, jarred, blended, and refined foods are all "verboten."

The Gerson recovery rate is estimated at 40 percent, a significant rate since 80 to 90 percent of all Gerson patients are admitted with "incurable" cancer. Treatment may take anywhere from three months to over one and one-half year, depending on the cancer involved. According to Charlotte Gerson Strauss, daughter of Dr. Max Gerson, however, improvement is usually seen within a few weeks after admittance.

Like other diets, the Gerson diet can be followed at home (see Dr. Max Gerson's book, *A Cancer Therapy—Results of Fifty Cases*), but since the program is extensive, including special supplements and organic foods such as calf's liver, plenty of determination is needed to stick with it.

It is my opinion that the only way to combat diseases such as cancer is to think and live holistically. In my opinion, it is foolish to expect one therapy to work for everyone. Disease has many causes, and what is detrimental to you may be harmless, perhaps even beneficial, to someone else. Therefore, I don't believe that we'll ever find *the* magic formula for cancer. Instead, we may recognize individuality and apply existing knowledge accordingly. It won't be simple, but then, what is?

I also think it is foolish to discard hope. If you strongly believe in a certain therapy or treatment, chances are you will benefit. By the same token, there seems little use in trying something you don't believe in.

Herbal therapy, for instance, is often ridiculed, especially when it comes to treating cancer. Yet treatment with chaparral tea, also called creosote bush (*Covillea mexicana*) has resulted in many recoveries. The Hoxsey treatment, for instance, is based on herbal therapy.

Laetrile, used by a number of unconventional cancer clinics worldwide, has received much publicity after Dr. Ernst Krebs, Jr. of San Francisco discovered that amygdalin, laetrile's active component, could assist pancreatic enzymes in destroying cancer without affecting healthy cells.

Laetrile, a plant product made from apricot pits, occurs naturally in many other seeds such as the kernels of peaches, bitter almonds, and apple seeds. Chemically speaking, laetrile is two parts sugar, one part benzaldehyde, and one part cyanide.

Dr. Robert Gibson of Ponca City, Oklahoma, along with other cancer specialists, uses laetrile in conjunction with vitamins A, C and E and enzymes, and with a salt-free, high-fiber nutritional plan similar to the Gerson diet. Dr. Gibson has treated numerous patients and says that for the terminally ill, laetrile is an effective pain reliever that, along with improved nutrition, often extends the patient's life expectancy.

Many cancer specialists admit, however, that laetrile is not consistently effective. Dr. Kenji Sakaguchi, one of Japan's top molecular biologists, indicates that this is due to the body's inefficiency to properly break down laetrile. In a nutshell, laetrile is not effective unless benzaldehyde is freed. According to the Japanese researcher, clinical studies demonstrated that patients treated with benzaldehyde had a 30% increase in recovery rate. Interestingly, similar results are reported by European cancer specialists who prescribe old-fashioned cancer diets that supply good amounts of benzaldehyde-rich foods such as berries.

Immunotherapy is used by a number of physicians, and although there is little evidence that specific vaccines will ever protect us from cancer, immunization is used to improve the body's defense or immune system which, in turn, aids recovery.

Although I generally don't endorse immunization, immunotherapy makes sense. A healthy immune system is the best protection against all diseases. When our immune system is down, we are susceptible to illness. Thus, I believe that the improvement of the immune system is vital no matter what the disease.

Disease is multicausal and the body's immune system can be depressed by malnutrition, acute and hidden allergies, emotional problems, infections, environmental pollutants including cigarettes and other chemical stressors. But to remove disease one has to remove the cause, and if this is not entirely possible one must recognize the immune system's need for support. Improve the immune system and the body can heal itself.

We also need to recognize individuality. The cancer patient who is constantly distressed about family or monetary problems will gain from nutritional therapy (because emotional distress induces specific nutritional needs), but unless his problems are solved, his immune system will suffer no matter how much nutritional support is given. By the same token, present cancer diets can never suit all cancer patients unless individual needs are recognized. Why, for instance, does one terminal cancer patient respond to one particular diet while another doesn't? I believe (and I must admit that I have no evidence for this yet) that food sensitivities may play a part. For example, if a patient has a slight, and therefore not recognized, allergy to certain fruits or vegetables, the best fresh food diet won't improve his condition unless the problem is recognized and dealt with. Since by some estimates 60% of the population suffers from unknown food intolerances or allergies, which definitely have a negative impact on the immune system, we may have to change our thinking and take yet a closer look at cancer patients. Why do some cancer patients have difficulties breaking down laetrile? Could that be linked to depressed enzyme activities as often found in food-sensitive patients? Admittedly, there are many questions to which I can provide no satisfactory answer, but perhaps if we pay more attention to the immune system, cancer will become less of a threat.

Interferon also supports the immune system. This natural anti-cancer agent is widely studied here and abroad. By 1980, the National Cancer Institute had invested 3.4 million dollars for interferon research with varying results. The catch is that interferon presently can only be made from large quantities of human white blood cells, resulting in astronomical prices. Interferon may be promising but so far few can afford treatment.

Hyperthermia is a relatively simple, old-time method of cancer treatment that is currently used and studied at Presbyterian Hospital in

Denver, Colorado and a few other institutions around the country.

Interestingly, this promising method dates to the nineteenth century when artificially-raised body temperatures of up to 105 degrees Fahrenheit effectively reduced cancer. While in the olden days, steam baths, hot tubs, and induced fever were used to fight off cancer with heat, modern hyperthermia employs microwaves, ultrasounds, and radiofrequency equipment. Today, hot beams are used, which when aimed directly at tumors, kill cancer cells but cause minimal or no danger to normal cells. The basic concept is that healthy cells withstand temperatures of up to 112 degrees Fahrenheit, while cancer cells are destroyed at approximately 107 degrees Fahrenheit.

If you are a cancer victim in search of an alternative cancer therapy, contact the Cancer Control Society, 2043 No. Bernedo Street, Los Angeles, Ca. 90027. (213) 663-7801.

HELPING CYSTIC FIBROSIS

This childhood disease, characterized by faulty digestion and extreme susceptibility to respiratory infections, is tied to a number of nutritional deficiencies. The digestive problems seen in the cystic fibrosis patient arise from the pancreas's inability to produce digestive enzymes, thus food remains undigested, causing persistent diarrhea and foul-smelling stools.

Because cystic fibrosis victims have an inability to break down and absorb fat, this excessive fat loss prevents absorption of the fat-soluble vitamins, particularly vitamins A and E. Autopsy studies of children who have died of the disease showed multiple signs of vitamin E deficiency. Lack of the B-vitamins, particularly B6, and the amino acid methionine has also been linked to the disease. Since pancreatic function is made worse by an excess of B1 and calcium, attention should be paid to establishing proper levels.

Supplementing the diet with pancreatic enzymes and lecithin aids the breakdown of fats, improving digestion and absorption. Nutritious foods such as yeast, wheat germ, liver, yogurt, vegetable juices such as carrot, dandelion, and white radish juice should be included in a diet that contains little or no saturated fats.

Certain herbs are known to stimulate pancreatic function, normally improving production of digestive enzymes. The following old-fashioned herbal tea mixture has been found to improve faulty digestion, resulting in better absorption of valuable nutrients.

Herbal Digestive Aid
(stimulates pancreatic function)

1 oz. blueberry leaves (*Vaccinium myrtillus*)
1 oz. dandelion root (*Taraxacum officinalis*)
1 oz. goldenseal rootstock (*Hydrastic canadensis*)
1 oz. marigold flowers (*Calendula officinalis*)
1 oz. nettle leaves (*Urtica dioica*)
1 oz. yarrow (*Achillea millefolium*)

Add 1 teaspoon herbal mixture to 1 cup cold water and bring to quick boil. Reduce from heat and steep for 3 minutes. Drink 1–2 quarts per day in small doses, depending on age.

In addition, prepare a sweet flag infusion by adding 1 teaspoon sweet flag rootstock (*Acorus calamus*) to ½ pint cold water. Soak overnight, heat up the following morning but do not boil. Strain and sip 1 teaspoon before and after meals, but do not take more than 6 teaspoons daily. Small children should take less, depending on age.

Meeting the patient's nutritional needs increases resistance to infectious diseases, thus preventing the need for antibiotics, which, incidentally, contribute to digestive problems and nutritional deficiencies.

AN UNCONVENTIONAL TREATMENT FOR CEREBRAL PALSY

The cause of this disease is considered to be the result of hemorrhaging in the brain or spinal cord and may be linked to deficiencies of the vitamins E and K. Cerebral palsy could, most likely, be prevented if expectant mothers would pay closer attention to their nutritional intake by eating liberal amounts of green, leafy vegetables (the main source of vitamin K) and wheat germ or other foods rich in vitamin E. Both of these vitamins are fat-soluble, requiring some fat intake and bile salts to metabolize them, thus pregnant mothers should not avoid all fats. When digestive problems are present as is often the case during pregnancy, a good digestive enzyme containing bile salts will help metabolize needed nutrients.

Newborn infants are generally deficient in vitamin K, and this is particularly the case when symptoms of malnutrition are observed in the mother. In such cases, the administration of 1 mg of vitamin K to the newborn infant, or 10 to 20 mg to the mother during labor could prevent cerebral palsy.

Those children suffering from the disease should eat a most wholesome diet and receive the vitamins E and B6 (5–50 mg daily, depending on age). Vitamin E has been found to be especially beneficial to CP patients, hence, 25 mg daily should be given during the first month of life and gradually be increased. A six-year-old should receive 50 mg, while a teenager would benefit from 100 to 200 mg daily.

Thirty years ago, Dr. Leo Spears of Spears Chiropractic Hospital in Denver stated that not all CP is caused by injury. Instead, he said, skull distortions which create pressure on the brain are the most frequent cause of the disease. After working with many young CP victims, Dr. Spears was convinced that distorted skull patterns, often the result of a difficult birth process which creates brain pressure rather than brain injury, is at fault in many cases.

Through "skull molding," Dr. Leo Spears simply normalized the distorted skull patterns of the very young and in many cases considerable improvement was evident. According to Dr. Spears, a child's skull reaches 90 percent of its growth and hardness during the first seven years of life, and the older the CP patient, the more difficult it is to correct skull distortions.

Unfortunately, the medical profession sees little merit in this natural treatment and has ignored it ever since; however, doctors at Spears Hospital and other chiropractors continue to work on a limited basis with cerebral palsy victims.

In the fall of 1979, I went to interview young Jeanie B. of Moro, Illinois, a cerebral palsy victim who had been admitted to Spears. Her story, told by mother and daughter, proved fascinating.

When Jeanie was 14 months old the disease was diagnosed and her mother was advised to institutionalize the youngster because the general prognosis was bad. Nobody believed that Jeanie would walk before the age of 8 or 9, or be able to communicate.

Jeanie, like other children before her, quickly responded to skull molding, also called cranial adjustments, and when I came to see her she was an energetic young lady who enjoyed running around the playground, riding a tricycle, and, despite a somewhat limited vocabulary, enjoyed talking like any 8- or 9-year-old.

I couldn't help but think of all the other cerebral palsy victims who might live fuller lives if only the treatment would be recognized. After all, what could they lose?

CENTURY-OLD REMEDIES THAT IMPROVE
PARKINSON'S DISEASE (*PARALYSIS AGITANS*)

This slowly progressive disorder of the central nervous system is characterized by tremor of resting muscles and by stiffness and slowness of movement. Typically, the victim displays masklike, waxen features, rhythmic tremor of the fingers; his posture is stooped and he walks as if he were about to collapse.

Chiropractic treatments, including physical therapy, help relieve symptoms. Peanut oil body rubs, says Dr. Harold Reilly, author of *The Edgar Cayce Handbook for Health Through Drugless Therapy*, aid patients suffering from all neuromuscular ailments. Dietary adjustments are necessary to prevent constipation, water accumulation, leg cramps, and other problems commonly associated with the disease.

Constipation commonly troubles patients, though a well-balanced high-fiber diet that includes adequate amounts of fresh fruits and vegetables, sprouts, nuts, and whole grains quickly improves digestion. If there is an additional need for bulk, fresh or dried figs, prunes, or other natural laxatives should be eaten frequently. Two to three tablespoons of bran sprinkled over soups, salads, yogurt, etc. restore normal bowel movements, quickly eliminating the need for pharmaceutical laxatives.

Other nutritional disorders are associated with the ailment. For example, studies demonstrated a relationship between a vitamin B6 deficiency and the disease, and when 10 to 200 milligrams of vitamin B6 (pyridoxine) were given daily, patients reported feeling stronger; they walked with a steadier gait and had better bladder control.

To improve bladder function, old-time herbal treatments produce excellent results. The herb uva ursi (see section on "Natural Diuretics" in Chapter 4), for instance, is one of the most effective, old-time remedies that continues to be endorsed by European medical doctors and other health care providers. The daily addition of up to 500 mg of the mineral magnesium also improves bladder function.

Since an alkaline environment encourages bacterial growth, vitamin C therapy and an adequate protein intake are needed to slightly acidify the urine to help prevent bladder infections and cystitis.

Generally, a well-balanced diet supplemented with the vitamins B6, E, and the mineral magnesium is most successful in the treatment of all nerve and muscle disorders including Parkinson's disease, cerebral palsy, epilepsy and other ailments where there is faulty transmission of nerve impulses to the muscular system. An ancient natural European therapy that stimulates the nervous system and improves circulation and muscle function is the dry brush massage. This simple self-treatment promotes elimination of toxic waste via the skin and promotes healing.

OLD-FASHIONED DRY BRUSH MASSAGE

All you need is a natural bristle brush with a handle long enough so you can reach all parts of your body. Starting with the soles of your feet,

brush vigorously, but gently. Use rotary motions and slowly move up-
wards toward the heart. After you've massaged all parts of your body, take
a hot shower until you are all warmed up, and then quickly rinse your
body with cold water. If you can't stand this "shock treatment," use a
warm shower instead, but rub yourself dry with a coarse towel.

Patients suffering from neuro-muscular diseases are easily overcome
by stress; therefore, emotional upsets should be avoided.

In short, *all* aspects need to be taken into account—because man is
a whole being and should always be treated as such.

SELECTING THE RIGHT KIND OF DOCTOR

I firmly believe that the best doctors are open-minded, inquisitive,
and unafraid of challenges. If you prefer such a doctor, ask around. One
of your friends, neighbors, or co-workers might know one. Check it out.

Call the doctor's office and find out as much about him and his
policies as possible. If everything sounds encouraging, make an appointment for a consultation during which you might want to ask the following useful eyeopeners:

1. Can nutrition help me?
2. Can herbal remedies be beneficial and perhaps replace drug
   therapy?
3. Do you inform patients about possible drug reactions, side effects, etc.?
4. Do you cooperate with other health care professions?
5. Would you refer me to a chiropractor, nutritionist, or any
   other nonmedical health care professional?
6. On an average, how much time do you spend with your patients?
7. Do you explain medical treatments?
8. Would you object to second and third opinions?
9. Will you try to make use of natural therapies whenever possible?
10. Can I object to being X-rayed?
11. If X-rays must be taken, do you shield patients' reproductive
    organs, and if possible, the thyroid?
12. Can I discuss and possibly object to some form of treatment
    without upsetting our relationship?

In case you are looking for a good chiropractor, dentist, or nutritionist, change the following questions to:

3. Do you check up on patients' drug intake?
4. Do you cooperate with medical doctors?
7. Do you explain your treatment methods?
9. Would you refer me to a medical doctor or any other health care professional if necessary?

If the doctor, nutritional consultant, or whatever type of health care professional you are consulting, answers "No," or "I don't know," more than twice, keep on looking.

ACCEPTING RESPONSIBILITIES

I can't say it often enough—drugs have spoiled us. Their "instant action" has made us expect instant relief. We detest pain, have grown unaccustomed to it.

Fever scares us, even though it is a healthy body response needed for healing. We expect doctors to perform instant miracles, and if they can't help, we are desperately lost without hope.

The trouble is, we have forgotten that our health is *our* primary responsibility. Doctors can assist us in getting well, but they cannot actually heal. Only our bodies can do that, provided we support their healing activities.

We have to change our thinking, depend more on ourselves and less on others. We have to learn responsibility, and once again listen to our elders who have much to offer.

Above all, we need to improve our resistance, because prevention is still our best strategy for combating diseases.

****

NATURAL HEALING GUIDE

Ailments, with Suggestions for Natural Treatments

(For more details see appropriate chapter.)

ADDISON'S DISEASE

Vitamins: B-complex, B2, B6, C, pantothenic acid; minerals: potassium; herbs: lemon balm, peppermint

ACNE VULGARIS

Vitamins: A, B-complex, and E (externally and internally); minerals: zinc; digestive enzymes; improve fiber intake; herbs: garlic, camomile steam facial; mud packs

ALLERGIES

Multivitamin, vitamins A and C, B-complex, pantothenic acid; amino acids, enzymes, lecithin, adrenal glandular, liver glandular; milk thistle

ANXIETY

B-complex, calcium-magnesium, vitamin D; brewer's yeast; borage, lemon balm, St. Johnswort, passionflower, valerian

ANEMIA, pernicious, megaloblastic, secondary

Iron, vitamin B12, C, folic acid, digestive enzymes containing betaine hydrochloric acid; liver or liver extract and other iron-rich foods, protein; beets; European vervain, juniper berries, oak bark, shave grass

ARTERIOSCLEROSIS

Multivitamin, vitamins C and E; chelated minerals and magnesium; artichoke juice; beets, garlic; reduced fat intake, increased fiber intake

ARTHRITIS

Multivitamin, calcium-magnesium, vitamin D, pantothenic acid; arnica flowers, angelica root, birch leaves, celery, oats, violet leaves; mud baths, oat bath

BACK PAIN

Vitamin C, calcium-magnesium; ice pack for acute pain; apply warmth for chronic pain

BRIGHT'S DISEASE

B-complex, choline, inositol, lecithin; alfalfa, black elder, goldenrod; celery, parsley

BRONCHITIS, ASTHMA

Vitamins A, C, B-complex; minerals: calcium, magnesium; hypoallergenic amino acids, enzymes; althaea, coltsfoot, fennel, island moss, licorice, lungwort, plantain, thyme; hot packs or diathermy

BRUISES

Vitamin C and rutin

BUERGER'S DISEASE

Vitamins: B6, B-complex, C and E (large doses), rutin; minerals: calcium, magnesium, potassium, lecithin; avoid nicotine; witch hazel (externally and internally), localized cold showers; arnica baths, yarrow baths (warm only); reduce meat intake; high-fiber foods to improve digestion; avoid animal fats and proteins

BURNING FEET

Vitamin B6, camomile foot bath, epsom salt foot bath

BURNS, to promote healing

Externally: vitamin E, oak bark infusion; internally: vitamin E, A, C and zinc; aloe vera, camomile

CALLUSES, CORNS, BUNIONS

Externally: vitamin E, celandine footbath, celandine juice; comfortable footware

COLDS, INFECTIONS

Vitamins: A, C, B-complex, multivitamin and -mineral, amino acids, enzymes, thymus nucleoprotein; althaea, eucalyptus, island moss, lungwort, thyme; gardencress, garlic

COLD EXTREMITIES

Vitamin C and E, niacin, RNA (ribo-nucleic acid); lemon balm, rosmarin

COLD SORES (Herpes Simplex)

Vitamin C, multivitamin and mineral, calcium, magnesium, zinc; lactobacillus acidophilus, amino acids especially lysine; garlic; burdock root, pokeweed; externally: vitamin E and zinc ointment for improved healing; avoid sweets and citrus fruits

COLICS

Multivitamin and mineral, calcium, magnesium, potassium; camomile, fennel, valerian

COLITIS

Vitamins A, C and E, bioflavonoids; magnesium, potassium; dietary fiber; althea (marshmallow root), camomile, peppermint; all cabbages; white cabbage juice

CONSTIPATION

Vitamin B-complex, digestive enzymes; beets, althea, fennel, linseed (flax), licorice, sassafras bran and/or high-fiber foods.

CUSHING'S DISEASE

Potassium in large doses

CYSTITIS

Vitamin C; increase protein intake, avoid citrus fruits; drink plenty of grape or cranberry juice to acidify urine, or take 1 teaspoon apple cider vinegar with water; birch leaves, dandelion, uva ursi

DIABETES

Vitamins: A, C, E, B-complex, B-6; chromium, magnesium, potassium, zinc; lecithin, pancreatic enzymes; artichoke, bilberry, cucumber, dandelion, fenugreek, juniper berries, kidney beans, yarrow; eat small meals frequently; reduce calorie intake if overweight

DIARRHEA

Potassium, multivitamin and mineral; activated charcoal (or burned toast), camomile, dried blueberries or unsweetened blueberry or blackberry juice; dietary fiber as absorbent

DIGESTION PROBLEMS

Multivitamin and mineral supplement, digestive enzymes; camomile, peppermint, yarrow

EARACHE

Vitamins A and C; garlic, camomile or potato poultice; apply few drops of vitamin E

EDEMA (water retention)

Vitamin D, B2, B12, pantothenic acid; calcium, potassium; beans, birch leaves, parsley, restharrow, uva ursi (temporarily)

EMPHYSEMA

Vitamins A, B-complex, folic acid, C; protein; lungwort; no smoking

EPILEPSY

Vitamin B6, B-complex, B2, pantothenic acid; magnesium; improve diet; reduce calcium intake; camomile, hops, lemon balm

ECZEMA

(See acne) vitamin C, zinc; garlic; poultices: comfrey, marigold, oak bark, walnut leaves; baths: camomile, oats, bran; avoid nicotine

EYE PROBLEMS

Vitamins: A, B2, B6, pantothenic acid, C; improve protein intake; red eyebright (external and internal)

FAST PULSE
Vitamin E, yarrow, valerian

FATIGUE
Vitamins C and E, B-complex, possibly iron (see anemia); amino acids; ginseng, lavender, lemon balm, rosmarin, (other herbs see anemia); improve diet, exercise

FEVER
Vitamin A and C; buck bean, bitterwort (yellow gentian), elderberries, linden flowers, willow bark; beet and carrot juice

FLATULENCE
Digestive enzymes containing betaine HCl, garlic, papaya; caraway, fennel seeds, sweet flag, peppermint, European centaury

GALLBLADDER PROBLEMS
Vitamins A, D, E; lecithin, acidophilus or plain yogurt; artichoke, dandelion, black radish, beets, peppermint; digestive enzymes containing bile; restrict fat intake, improve protein intake but prevent acidosis

GASTRITIS
Vitamin B-complex, digestive enzymes; camomile, fennel, European centaury; light meals; no caffeine, alcohol or other stimulants

GOITER, toxic
Vitamins: B-complex, B6, C, E, potassium iodide or kelp; eliminate peanuts, untoasted soyflower, and all vegetables of the cabbage family

GOUT
Multivitamin and mineral supplement, potassium; reduce meat intake; cherry juice, unsweetened; pimpernel, birch leaves; hot oatstraw bath, hot potato poultice

HALITOSIS (bad breath)
Multivitamin and mineral supplement, digestive enzymes containing betaine Hcl, increase fiber intake; chew dill seeds (other herbs, see flatulence)

HAYFEVER, sinusitis (see colds)
Vitamins: A and C, B-complex, pollen (also see allergy), camomile vapor bath

HEMORRHOIDS
Vitamin E (internally and externally), multivitamin, zinc, dietary fiber;

fennel, yarrow, milk thistle; camomile sitz bath; zinc ointment (externally)

HEPATITIS

B-complex, choline, pantothenic acid, vitamins C and E, B-complex, B6, pantothenic acid; lecithin; artichoke juice; black radish, dandelion, milk thistle; improve protein intake but prevent acidosis, reduce fat intake; eat small meals frequently

HYPERACTIVITY

Multivitamin, B-complex (high doses), rutin, calcium-magnesium, potassium; camomile, fennel, lemon balm, valerian; avoid all food colorings and flavorings; lemon balm or camomile bath

HYPERTENSION (high blood pressure)

Garlic, hawthorn, lemon balm, milk thistle, mistletoe, digestive enzymes; restrict salt and animal proteins; no stimulants, alcohol or nicotine; small meals; juices, moderate exercise

HYPOGLYCEMIA

Multivitamin and mineral, vitamins C and E, B-complex, pantothenic acid; potassium; beets, milk thistle; small meals, amino acids, enzymes

HYPOTENSION (low blood pressure)

B-complex, multivitamin, adrenal glandular; hawthorn, ginseng, rosmarin; exercise

HYPOTHYROIDISM

Multivitamin and mineral, vitamins C, E, B-complex; kelp (natural source of iodine); lecithin, digestive enzymes, amino acids, thyroid glandular; bayberry, milk thistle, myrrh, black cohosh

INDIGESTION

B-complex, digestive enzymes, camomile, peppermint

IMPETIGO

Vitamins A and E (internally and externally), camomile bath; garlic oil (external application)

INSOMNIA

Vitamin B6, calcium-magnesium, potassium, tryptophan; camomile, lemon balm, hawthorn, passion flower, primrose, valerian; hot camomile bath

KIDNEY STONES

Vitamin A and C; chelated magnesium; pimpernel tea; grape juice, cranberry juice; warm shave grass or oat straw bath

LARYNGITIS

Vitamins A, C, B-complex; zinc; althea root, coltsfoot, mullein, pimpernel; hot milk and honey; hot camomile gargle

LEG CRAMPS

Vitamin B6, pantothenic acid; calcium, magnesium, potassium silica; lemon balm, hops, shave grass, valerian; increase vegetable oil intake

LIVER AILMENTS (see hepatitis)

LIVER SPOTS

Vitamin E; dandelion root

LUPUS ERYTHEMATOSUS

Multivitamin and mineral, vitamin E, pantothenic acid, PABA (external and internal); carrot juice

MENSTRUAL CRAMPS

Vitamin D, calcium, magnesium; beets, camomile, lady's mantle, shepherd's purse, silverweed, St. Johnswort, yarrow

MENSTRUATION, irregular or lack of

Multivitamin and mineral supplement, vitamin C, B-complex, B12, folic acid, E, calcium, magnesium; amino acids, herbs (see menstrual cramps). Problems are commonly associated with malnutrition and/or underweight

MENOPAUSE

Multivitamin and mineral supplement, vitamins D, E, B-complex, pantothenic acid; calcium, magnesium; amino acids; lemon balm, hawthorn, hops, lady's mantle, motherwort, sarsaparilla, shepherd's purse

MULTIPLE SCLEROSIS

Vitamin B-complex, B6, pantothenic acid, vitamin E; chelated minerals; digestive enzymes; lecithin; polyunsaturated fats (use peanut, safflower, and sunflower oils), eliminate saturated fats (animal fats); largely vegetarian diet; primrose

MUSCLE STIFFNESS (after heavy exercise)

Hot lemon balm or rosmarin bath

MUSCLE WEAKNESS

Vitamin B6, potassium, amino acids

MUSCULAR DYSTROPHIES

Vitamins, A, B6 and E; amino acids; no refined foods

MYASTHENIA GRAVIS

Multivitamin and mineral supplement, B-complex, vitamins C and E; manganese, potassium; lecithin; arachidonic acid (found in peanuts and peanut oil); improve protein (amino acid) intake; eat wholesome foods only

NASAL CATARRH

Vitamins A, C, B-complex; eucalyptus oil vapor bath (also see bronchitis)

NAUSEA and vomiting

Vitamin B6, magnesium; artichoke, peppermint

NEPHRITIS

Multivitamin and mineral, vitamins A, C and E (also see Bright's disease)

NERVOUSNESS (see anxiety)

NEURALGIA, NEURITIS

Multivitamin and mineral, B-complex, B1, B2, B6, B12, pantothenic acid; calcium; lecithin; dietary fiber; brewer's yeast; liver; no refined carbohydrates; no alcohol; hops, lemon balm, peppermint, valerian

NIGHT SWEAT

Calcium carbonate, hops, sage

OSTEOPOROSIS

Vitamin D, calcium, magnesium; lecithin, digestive enzymes containing HCl

PANCREATITIS

Vitamins B6, E; pancreatic enzymes; amino acids; acidophilus; camomile

PARALYSIS

Vitamins B1, B2, B6, potassium; lemon balm

PHLEBITIS

Multivitamin and mineral supplement, B-complex, vitamins C and E; lecithin; rue (for other herbs, see Buerger's disease)

POISON IVY

Witch hazel, gum plant; very hot shower or epsom salt bath

PROSTATE PROBLEMS

Multivitamin and mineral supplement, vitamins A, E, B6, C, and pantothenic acid; zinc; pumpkin seeds

SICKLE CELL ANEMIA

Vitamins C and E, zinc; decrease iron intake (serum iron often high), shave grass

SINUSITIS

(See colds, infections)

SPRUE

B-complex, folic acid; all green vegetables; camomile/peppermint tea

STINGS, BITES

Vitamin C, B6, papain (externally)

STREP THROAT

Vitamins A and C, B-complex; garlic, thyme, Iceland moss

STRETCH MARKS

Vitamin B-complex, pantothenic acid, E (externally and internally), exercise

SUNBURNS

PABA, zinc, externally: aloe vera, baking soda/cornstarch mixture

TASTE, loss of

Multivitamin and mineral supplement, vitamin B6, zinc; shave grass

TENNIS ELBOW (trick knee, etc.)

Vitamin C, multivitamin and mineral, manganese

ULCERS, peptic, jejenum, duodenum

Vitamins A, E, B-complex; camomile, papaya; white cabbage juice; eat small meals frequently; avoid all stimulants; avoid stress; reduce fat and meat intake

URINARY INFECTIONS

Vitamins A, C, E, B-complex; garlic, cranberry and grape juice, uva ursi

VAGINAL YEAST INFECTION (vaginitis)

Vitamins A, C, B-complex, high potency, zinc; acidophilus; camomile sitz bath; no alkaline foods (citrus fruits, etc.)

VARICOSE VEINS

(See Buerger's disease)

VITILIGO

PABA, B-complex; liver; milk thistle

WARTS

Vitamin A and E (useful externally and internally); apply plain white chalk several times daily

WORMS, intestinal

Vitamins A, B-complex, multivitamin and mineral; carrot juice, garlic, pumpkin seeds; improve diet

Bibliography

RECOMMENDED READINGS

Airola, Paavo, Ph.D., N.D. *How to Get Well.* Phoenix, Arizona: Health Plus, Publ., 1980.

————. *How to Keep Slim, Healthy and Young with Juice Fasting.* Phoenix, Arizona: Health Plus Publ., 1971.

Barnes, Broda O., M.D. and Galton Lawrence. *Hypothyroidism, The Unsuspected Illness.* Crowell, 1976.

Bircher-Benner. *Nutrition Plan for Raw Food and Juices.* Nash Publ., 1972.

Bricklin, Mark. *The Practical Encyclopedia of Natural Healing.* Rodale Press, 1980.

Cheraskin, E., M.D., D.M.D.; Ringsdorf, W.M. Jr. *Preventive Medicine, A Study in Strategy.* Keats Publ., 1973.

Cheraskin, E., M.D., D.M.D.; Ringsdorf, W.M., Jr., D.M.D.; Clark, J.W., D.D.S. *Diet and Disease.* Keats, 1968.

Clark, Linda. *Handbook of Natural Remedies for Common Ailments.* Connecticut: Devin-Adair, 1976.

Donsbach, Kurt, Ph.D. *Nutrition in Action.* Intern. Institute of Natural Health Sciences, Inc., 1977.

Editors of Runner's World Magazine. *The Complete Runner.* Avon, 1974.

Fredericks, Carlton, Ph.D. *New and Complete Nutrition Handbook.* International Institute of Natural Health Sciences, Ca., 1964.

Gerson, Max. M.D. *A Cancer Therapy/50 Case Histories.* Rev., Bonita, California: Gerson Inst., 1956.

Graedon, Joe. *The People's Pharmacy.* Avon Books, 1976.

Grieve, M. *A Modern Herbal.* Volumes I and II. Dover Publ., 1971.

Heinerman, John. *Science of Herbal Medicine.* Utah: By-World, 1979.

Hodges, Robert E., M.D. *Nutrition in Medical Practice.* Saunders Co., 1980.

Hutchens, Alma R. *Indian Herbology of North America.* Ontario, Canada: Merco, 1973.

Kloss, Jethro. *Back to Eden.* Woodbridge Press, 1975.

Krochmal, Arnold and Connie. *A Guide to Medicinal Plants of the United States.* Quadrangle, 1975.

Kugler, Hans, Ph.D. *Dr. Kugler's Seven Keys to a Longer Life.* New York: Stein and Day, 1978.

Kunz-Bircher, Ruth. *The Bircher-Benner Health Guide.* Woodbridge Press Publ., 1980.

Lust, John B., N.D., D.B.M. *The Herb Book.* Bantam Book, 1974.

Matthews, Bryan. *Multiple Sclerosis.* Oxford, England: Oxford University Press, 1978.

Mendelsohn, Robert, S., M.D. *Male Practice.* Chicago: Contemporary Books, 1981.

————. *Medical Heretic.* ————, 1980.

Miller, Lois Mattox; Thomson, Susan W. *Handbook of First Aid.* Reader's Digest Assn., 1975.

Moss, Ralph, W. *The Cancer Syndrome.* New York: Grove Press, 1980.

Null, Gary. *The New Vegetarian.* New York: W. Morrow & Co., 1978.

Passwater, Richard, Ph.D. *Supernutrition for Healthy Hearts.* Jove Publ., 1977.

Pfeiffer, Carl, C., M.D., Ph.D. *Mental and Elemental Nutrients.* Keats Publ., 1975.

Reilly, Harold; Hagy Brod, Ruth. *The Edgar Cayce Handbook for Health Through Drugless Therapy.* Macmillan, 1975.

Reuben, David, M.D. *The Save Your Life Diet.* New York: Random House, 1975.

Robinson, Corinne, H. *Normal and Therapeutic Nutrition.* New York: Macmillan, 1972.

Secretary, Heath, Education and Welfare. *Marihuana and Health.* DHEW Publ. No. (ADM) 77–443, 1977.

Selye, Hans, M.D. *Stress Without Distress.* Signet, 1975.

Simmonite-Culpeper. *Herbal Remedies.* Foulsham & Co., 1957.

Simmonton, O. Carl, M.D.; Matthews-Simmonton, Creighton, James. *Getting Well Again.* New York: St. Martin's Press, 1978.

Sportelli, Louis, D.C. *Introduction to Chiropractic.* Sportelli, 1978.

Strauss, R.H., M.D. *Sports Medicine and Physiology.* Saunders, 1979.

Verrett, Jacqueline; Carper, Jean. *Eating May Be Hazardous to Your Health.* Anchor Books, 1978.

Williams, Roger, J., Ph.D. *Nutrition Against Disease.* New York: Pitman Publ., 1971.

_____. *Nutrition in a Nutshell.* Doubleday, Inc., 1962.

_____. *The Wonderful World Within You.* Bantam Books, 1977.

GERMAN PUBLICATIONS

Furlenmeier, M., M.D. *Wunderwelt der Heilpflanzen.* Eltville/Rhein: Rheingauer Verlag, 1978.

Goerz, Heinz. *Gesundheit durch Heilkraeuter.* Wiesbaden: W. Moeller Verlag, 1974.

Lindt, Inge. *Naturheilkunde.* Buch und Zeit Verlag, Koeln, 1977.

Mar, Lisa; Kleine, H.O., M.D. *Krebsdiät.* Weil der Stadt: W. Haedecke Verlag, 1965.

Schauenberg, P.; Paris, F. *Heilpflanzen BLV Bestimmungsbuch.* Muenchen: BLV Verlag, 1978.

Stage, Wolfgang, M.D. *Das Kneipp Taschenbuch.* Frankfurt: Ullstein, 1968.

Thomson, W.A., M.D., et al. *Heilpflanzen und ihre Kraefte.* Lingen, Koeln, 1978.

Treben, Maria. *Gesundheit aus der Apotheke Gottes.* Steyr, Austria: Ennsthaler Verlag, 1980.

Index